Subconscious Medicine

I0130039

DEE TWENTYMAN

ISBN: 1927677785

ISBN-13-9781927677780

DEE TWENTYMAN

Dedication

This book is for all the people who experience Pain on a daily basis, and believe there is an alternative to drugs in order to become well.

CONTENTS

Acknowledgements

· I would like to thank my teachers both at school and university for creating the enjoyment I have in learning about the mind and the body.

· To everyone at the Croft Academy where I began my journey into a career as a Hypnotherapist.

· To Terence Watts for further learning and instilling the belief in my own knowledge and skills.

· To Ron Eslinger, for cementing my desire to specialise in the treatment of pain.

· To Mike Berry, for editing and formatting this book and his ongoing support and patience at my lack of computer skills, when I ring up again and say *'I need help, I've forgotten what you told me!'*

· To Darren Eden for teaching me to work with my intuition and giving me the belief that I should write a book.

· To everyone who has encouraged me, and supported me. Last but by no means least, to the clients who have put their faith in me, and placed themselves in my hands, as the person who teaches them to help themselves. I wish you all a peaceful mind and body.

Foreword

Life as we know it in the West is one in which we expect an instant response to much of what ails us. We live in a *'Pill for all Ills'* mentality. However, some of these instant cures have a whole host of side effects that can often be far worse than the initial illness. Our ancestors relied on their own inner resources, the same resources that each and every human being is born with. Many of our brothers and sisters in other cultures around the world are still relying on these methods to ease pain in their bodies, with huge success.

Subconscious Medicine(tm) by Dee Twentyman is intended to help you understand the mind-body connection to pain. It is this connection that you can tap into and use, to achieve more comfort in your daily life, and free yourself from Chronic Pain. When I am in pain, like many people I take a painkiller, when that doesn't work I may take something else, but then if I am still in pain, I am left with no where to go, I may have to 'suffer'. The techniques discussed in this book from Dee's self-help pain management programme, now give people like you and I somewhere to go when the drugs don't work. When you practice them, and explore the power of your unique mind, you are giving yourself a gift that will last a lifetime and one you can pass on to others. This book will encourage you to challenge your beliefs, about what is possible for you.

In this book:

*You will explore the interconnections of your beliefs, expectations, fears, and actions that reinforce or reduce pain sensations in your body.

*You will learn that as you practice the techniques and hone your skills, you will start to become more in control of your thoughts, feelings and actions, and all this feeds your confidence in your abilities to heal yourself, and strengthen your beliefs in the process.

*You will have a deeper understanding of how your brain registers pain and what you can do to harness the power of your mind.

*You will be given several FREE bonuses to get you started on this new journey of a peaceful mind and body.

I am delighted to write the foreword to Subconscious Medicine(tm), written by an excellent therapist and a specialist in the use of these techniques that will surely bring you the relief you have been looking for.

Raymond Aaron
New York Times Best Selling Author of
Chicken Soup for the Parents Soul.

Introduction

One of the first things to understand about pain; is that it is a subjective experience. This means that your experience is unique to you, and there is no other person who will feel pain or experience pain in exactly the same way that you will. The second thing to understand is that there is, as yet, no scientific way of measuring the experience of pain in an objective way. There is no way of measuring the tension or the discomfort that anyone of us experiences in our bodies.

When asked to describe our pain to others, we often find it difficult to get across exactly how that pain feels. We use words such as throbbing, knawing, gripping, etc. and yet your experience of these words, will not be the same as someone else.

As well as the pain, there will be other factors that add to or diminish the pain. Your experience of pain isn't simply a sensation, or a feeling you have due to the physical damage to your organs, bones or tissues. Pain is an experience that also includes emotions, and thoughts and physical sensations. Our thoughts and emotional connections can and do affect the level of pain we experience. Due to this interconnectedness, it is more than possible to change your experience of pain, using the power of your thoughts, and harnessing your belief system in the most positive and amazing way.

Not only can you reduce the pain, you can often eliminate it altogether. This book will help you to gain a better understanding of this Mind-Body Connection so that you can begin to use it effectively to manage Chronic Pain. It has also been used to help women in childbirth have a far more comfortable birthing experience.

Another remarkable phenomenon of how the mind and body connection works with pain sensations is called Phantom Limb Pain. The way our bodies' cells respond and interact, means pain can also be felt when the affected body part or limb is no longer there. Many amputees experience Phantom Limb pain.

The sensations, interpreted as pain, can be felt for years after the limb is removed. These are memories and signals from the part of our brain that affects our emotions and thoughts.

The person knew there was an arm or a leg there; they still carry an emotional attachment to that limb. Whether that attachment is a longing for it to be part of them again, even with the pain that went with it, or whether we have a profound memory of the pain that was there. This clearly demonstrates how complete, but also how interconnected the mind and the body are. There is also the theory that our 'mind' and 'memory' are not just a part of our brain, but actually a part of every cell in our body.

In order to look at how you, and indeed every one of us, can help ourselves to experience comfort, this book will take a brief look at some theories of how the cells in our body are organised and controlled. Once we have an understanding of this, we will be more able to believe, and understand that we can truly alter the perception of pain when it happens.

This book will look relatively simply at genetics and how we can even work with our minds to alter the outcomes of negative suggestions given to us by the medical profession.

I will provide evidence from scientists and neuro physicists, biologists and GP's and surgeons throughout the years, highlighting cases that have helped to generate more investigation and research in this area. We look also at the power of our expectations, our powerful belief system, and cultural differences, religious and spiritual traditions that create different outcomes to pain.

The power of music too, can alter our experiences. The book also addresses the power of positive relationships, holding on to pain, and so much more.

There have been numerous experiments and research projects into how our body and mind interprets pain, and I will be relating to these throughout this easy to read and understand book. As more and more research and scientific studies take place, many more people within the scientific and medical professions are beginning to unravel some of the older theories, and the results have been astonishing.

Many of these older theories have been turned on their heads. No doubt many more theories will fall by the wayside in coming years. Some astonishing results about mind power have gone back to the 1800's and yet we still rely heavily upon drug treatments to alleviate whatever afflicts us.

Much of this is due to the medical model of care that we have in the West. Let's not also forget the financial grip of the powerful drug companies. It's safe to say that if the medical profession were to teach patients to harness the power of their own mind, based on their findings, then it is very easy to see the immense impact this would have on the profits of the drug companies.

Even so, more and more people are moving towards self-help, complementary and alternative treatments, for all the things that the human being experiences. Once again, some astounding results and 'cures' have been reported.

This book will help you to understand the mind-body connection to pain, and it also offers you the opportunity to learn and practice the powerful benefits of hypnosis and meditation to control chronic pain, with the use of my Self-Help pain management programme.

Pain-management using hypnosis has a long history, which is backed up by empirical research. More and more people are using hypnosis and meditation in medical practice all over the world.

As we take a more holistic approach to patient care, it is likely to grow even more in the years to come. Throughout this book I will be talking about the use of hypnosis and meditation, both as additions to traditional medication, and also as an alternative for some people.

Many people have either intolerance to, or allergies to pain killing drugs, and for those people in particular, this book will show how using the powerful mind, they can encourage the release of the body's own powerful anaesthetic and analgesic chemicals, and create feelings of comfort and well-being.

Understanding the mind-body connection, and practicing daily the techniques and strategies included as bonuses with this book, will show you that this is a viable alternative to painkilling medication. It can help reduce the use of anti-nociceptive drugs, reducing the risk of tolerance and dependence. So let's now take a look at the amazing powerful effects of mind over matter.

1. Hypnosis and Healing

There are many ways in which we can use our mind to alter how we feel. It's likely that you have heard of meditation, visualisation, positive thinking, intuitive guidance, affirmations, and focus to name a few. The most controversial and the most widely misunderstood way of using our mind power, in ways that are not only helpful but healing, is hypnosis. Many people are still quite suspicious and afraid of hypnosis, and this may even be you. Many people who have used hypnosis or thought about using it for health, or any emotional reason, will have unique experiences, expectations and perceptions of its power.

Hypnosis has been around for many years and that is part of another chapter. What I want you to understand about hypnosis and healing here, is that you are not a passive recipient of the process, where a therapist will sit you down, ask you to close your eyes, speak soft words of encouragement, which may or may not be physically heard, and your problems are instantly solved. Hypnosis is a process whereby you, as the client, begin to put into action the strategies and techniques suggested, and begin to notice welcome positive changes in your feelings, and sense of well-being. In effect it needs your active participation.

Brain Wave States

The hypnotic state is a normal and natural state of the human experience. We enter hypnosis many times during our everyday life. It is simply an altered state of awareness. During the day our brain waves move through various cycles or speed. During these altered cycles we are open to learning, conditioning, logical-reasoning and dreaming. There are two brainwave cycles that have been identified, as the optimum brain activity to take onboard new insights that can be beneficial, and alter how you think and feel about certain things. A short and simple explanation will help you understand why a hypnotherapist helps you, with your full participation, to enter these brainwave states.

Our brains have four main types of brain-waves; these can be measured by EEG readings. This is where electrodes are painlessly, attached to your scalp, and the readings are measured on the Encephalograph. Each type of brain wave has specific frequencies (more about frequencies in a short while) which then produce certain effects.

Beta Brain Waves operate at 13-30 cycles per second. This is the fastest brainwave cycle and we experience this when we are in the most intense state of alertness. This brainwave state is used when we are operating from our maximum mind power. All five external senses are active, our logical mind is active; it is essentially our logical everyday 'thinking' state.

Alpha Brain Waves operate at 8 to 12 cycles per second. This brain wave indicates a relaxed state of mind. It is a state of relaxed alertness, good for inspiration and learning facts fast. It's a meditative mind. In this state you can tap into internal "antenna" like qualities; capable of visions, powerful ideas, mindless creation of the incredible, internal feelings & sensations.

Theta Brain Waves operate at 4 to 8 cycles per second. This is where we experience deep meditation, deep inward thought. This is associated with life-like imagination. A high state of mental concentration; It's your magical mind, where you have internal pictures / visualisations. You use your Intuition, and inner guidance. During this state you can gain access to unconscious material. It is also a state of dreaming.

Delta Brain Waves operate at 0.5 to 4 cycles per second. This is deep dreamless sleep, deep relaxation, where you experience a state of oneness. It's associated with pure being & will. Various studies have shown that learning in the 'Alpha State' enhances our performance, but learning is more than just absorbing information. It has been found that changing the state of mind to operate in Beta, Alpha and Theta is most likely to produce the best learning, cognition and creativity, while also staying in a relaxed state of mind.

From birth to four years, babies' brains operate in the delta state, with brain waves running below 4 cycles per second. In adults, this level of brain wave activity is experienced in the deepest levels of sleep.

From four to seven years old, children operate in theta state, with brain waves running between four and seven cycles per second. In adults, this level of brain wave activity is experienced during sleep and also during states of fear when the body goes into a 'fight or flight' response. This is a powerful level from which to initiate change. In this state, we only need one or two experiences of learning to change behaviour.

From the ages seven to fourteen years, children live in the alpha state of 7 - 14 cycles per second. In adults, this is associated with light sleep, meditation, or eyes-closed relaxation. At this level, effective learning can take place after about 21 repetitions. Practice a new behaviour for 21 consecutive days, and that behaviour becomes a habit. Research has shown that strong levels of physical healing can take place when the brain is operating at 10 cycles per second.

From puberty through adulthood, the brain operates in the beta state, 14 - 21 cycles per second. This is experienced in the normal state of eyes open, awake and alert. In this state it may take many thousands of repetitions to learn a new behaviour. To create significant change in our lives at this level takes a great deal of time and effort.

You can probably now see how the Alpha and Theta brainwave states are the ones used by hypnotherapists to help you access your powerful inner resources; Resources that you can use to help your body heal. You may also now understand how we have picked up our behaviours, beliefs, and opinions, if we basically live in an hypnotic state from birth to puberty. This is another reason why therapists often ask about your childhood, because it's very likely that whatever issues you have, are the result of some childhood experience.

Delta & Theta brain waves are very good for health in general, and are normally obtained by sleep. But for students or others who work too hard, accessing them at the same time as other brain waves is rejuvenating. It's interesting to look at what happens within the body when we experience the various brainwave states.

NB. Frequencies in italics cover more than one brain wave frequency range. The release of endorphins by the delta brainwave can also be achieved by meditation, runners-high, and breathing exercises. (NLPLearningsystems.com)

Delta Brain Waves (0.5Hz to 4Hz)

0.5 Hz - Relaxation, helps soothe headaches

0.5 - 1.5 Hz - Pain relief; Endorphin release

0.9 Hz - Euphoric feeling

1 Hz - Wellbeing. Harmony and balance

2.5 Hz - Production of endogenous opiates (pain killers, reduce anxiety)

2.5 Hz - Relieves migraine pain. Produces endogenous opiates

3.4 Hz - Helps achieve restful sleep

3.5 Hz - Feeling of unity with everything. Whole being regeneration

3.9 Hz - Self renewal, enhanced inner awareness

4.0 Hz - Encephalin release for reduced stress

4.0 Hz - Allows brain to produce encephalin, all natural pain killer

4.0 Hz - Full memory scanning. Releases encephalin

4.0 Hz - Vital for memory and learning. Problem solving, object naming

1 - 3 Hz - Profound relaxation; restorative sleep; Tranquility and peace

Theta Brain Waves (4Hz to 8 Hz)

4.5 Hz - Brings about Shamanic/Tibetan state of consciousness, Tibetan chants.

4.9 Hz - Induce relaxation and deeper sleep

4.9 Hz - Introspection. Relaxation, meditation

5 Hz - Reduces sleep required. Theta replaces need for extensive dreaming

5.35 Hz - Allows relaxing breathing, free and efficient

5.5 Hz - Inner guidance, intuition

6.5 Hz - Centre of Theta frequency. Activates creative frontal lobe

7.5 Hz - Activates creative thought for art, invention, music. Problem solving

7.5 Hz - Ease of overcoming troublesome issues

7.83 Hz - Schumann earth resonance. Grounding, meditative, leaves you revitalized

3 - 8 Hz - Deep relaxation, meditation; Lucid dreaming

3 - 8 Hz - Increased memory, focus, creativity

4 - 7 Hz - Profound inner peace, emotional healing; lowers mental fatigue.

4 - 7 Hz - Deep meditation; near-sleep brainwaves.

Alpha brain waves (8Hz to 12Hz)

8- 10 Hz Super-learning new information; memorization; not comprehension.

8.22 Hz - Associated with the mouth. Brings creativity

10 Hz - Enhanced serotonin release. Mood elevation, arousal, stimulant

10 Hz - Provides relief from lost sleep, improves general mood

10 Hz - Mood elevator. Used to dramatically reduce headaches

10 Hz - Clarity, subconscious correlation. Releases serotonin

11 Hz - Relaxed yet awake state

12 Hz - Centering, mental stability.

11 - 14 Hz - Increased focus and awareness

12 - 14 Hz - Learning frequency, good for absorbing information passively

Beta brain waves (13Hz to 30Hz)

14 Hz – Awakeness; alert; Concentration on tasks; Focusing; vitality.

16 Hz - Bottom of hearing range. Releases oxygen/calcium into cells

12 - 15 Hz - Relaxed focus, improved attentive abilities

13 - 27 Hz - Promotes focused attention toward external stimuli

13 - 30 Hz - Problem solving, conscious thinking

18-24 Hz — Euphoria, can result in headaches, anxiety.

Each and every one of us is capable of accessing these brain waves and harnessing their power. Many scientific studies have been conducted over the last 50 or so years, to help us understand more about how our mind and bodies react to stimuli, and how exactly this happens. There have been some surprising and exciting findings, and more and more amazing discoveries are yet to be brought to our attention in the years to come, I'm sure.

2. Genetics

Within our bodies we have trillions of cells, and inside each cell is information from our DNA (Deoxyribonucleic acid). This information contains the complete set of instructions for how each cell behaves, depending on which type of cell it is. The information dictates, among other things, the life span of each cell, its maturity, its function and behaviour and even when that cell dies. Scientists have studied genetics for years and we now understand that genes are the units of our DNA, and this DNA is coiled to form something called chromosomes. We get one set of chromosomes from our mothers, and the other set from our fathers.

Each one of our cells has a nucleus, except for mature red blood cells, and the DNA in each chromosome makes up many genes, this DNA information is like a secret code. It has taken scientists many years to unravel the secret of our DNA, and there are still large sequences to this code that remain unknown. Our cells produce protein and enzymes; these are the chemical messengers within our cells produced by the gene being copied. The human genome project was completed in 2003 where almost 13000 genes were mapped within the body.

The Medical Model

It is because of the research and experiments over many, many years, that we have the Medical Model of care and treatment in the West. This Medical Model states that we human beings are biochemical machines, and that we are genetically controlled. What this suggests, is that if we have a weakness, or a strength in a part of our body which we say it is due to our heredity. If we have an intellectual strength in one area, if we are artistic or mentally defective, it is often presumed that these are genetically pre-programmed at our conception, and that they are part of us, part of our genetic coding, and therefore cannot be changed.

However, with this way of thinking, and with the belief in this philosophy, we severely limit ourselves. It stops us from understanding the huge capacity of our body to heal itself and it then fosters the perception that there is no way that the body can heal itself. This automatically means we revert to the 'medicine' to heal us. We contact our GP to write us a prescription for the pills or the potions.

It is true that genes do play a huge role within our body. However, to what extent? If genes do have the 'control' over the body as the medical model suggests, how then do we explain the accounts of amazing results over lethal genetic diseases that are cured using hypnosis? I will share one such example of this in the next chapter. There has to be something else going on; something much more profound, and indeed there is.

Environment

It is now widely recognised that our environment, our perception of it, and how we interpret it, has a direct control on the activity of our genes. This perception is not only how we, as complete human beings, respond to the environment, there is also the way that environmental signals are perceived by individual cells. Cells do become aware of a stimulus from its environment, such as oxygen, toxins, light etc. and it then has a behaviour response.

Human beings are complex organisms; we evolved from the earlier single cell life forms over millions of years. As we evolved, our brains developed something called the limbic system, this system converts signals into sensations, and they reach the conscious mind where they are then experienced as emotions.

What and Where is the mind?

This is going to be quite interesting to answer, because even scientists, biologists and physicists, with more academic knowledge and understanding than I have, still have no definitive answer to this question. What I aim to do, is to put the information I have gained from years of study, into an easy to understand format, so that you can put it into context of why and how to use your mind power to help relieve pain. This book is about the mind and body connection to pain and in order to fully understand this, we are going to shed further light on where the mind-body connection comes from.

Many people think that the mind is the brain. Many others think that the brain is the mind. Both are incorrect. For years now, we have been told that the mind is somewhere within the brain. If you imagine that your brain is like a galaxy in outer space, then your mind is in that galaxy. However, further in this chapter we will look at other research that offers another theory.

What we do now know, is that the mind operates from mental, emotional and physical responses to stimuli. The 'mental process', or 'thinking' in other words, involves pathways called 'neural pathways' along which messages travel. They pass on these messages via electrical and chemical processes. Our brain is a mass of electrical energy and hormones, and other biochemicals make up the chemical component of energy in our brain.

The emotional process is set off by our memories. We then get a hormonal response from our body, either feel good hormones such as:

- Serotonin which regulates our mood, prevents depression and makes you feel happy. Serotonin is released by exposure to sunlight, and by eating foods rich in carbohydrates and by exercising.
- Endorphins; these can make you feel good, reduce your anxiety and your sensitivity to pain. Endorphins are also released by spending time exercising.
- Dopamine; this helps you to feel mentally alert.
- Phenylethamine; this is the hormone that results in the feelings we get in the early stages of a relationship. It is also contained in Cocoa beans, which explains a little why eating chocolate gives us the feel good factor.
- Gherlin; is a hormone that reduces stress and can help you become more relaxed.

We also have other hormones that are released when we feel anxious or some other negative emotion. Such as: Adrenaline, Norepinephrine, and Cortisol.

- Adrenaline is responsible for the immediate reactions we feel when we become stressed.
- Norepinephrine is another hormone released by the adrenal glands and helps you to focus, and it helps move the blood flow to where it is needed, usually to the muscles so that you can flee the scene.
- Finally, Cortisol is named the Stress hormone and takes a little longer to be released, once another part of your brain, called the amygdala, recognises that there is a threat.

You can now see how, what we think and feel has an automatic physical response and this is where we get the mind and body connection. It's true to say that we really cannot separate the mind and the body.

Everything we think has an effect on our body, as does our emotions. The cells of our body have memories that can, if triggered by something, take us right back to the original event as if it were yesterday.

Do Cells have Memory?

The miracle that is our body has an intelligence that knows no bounds. Your body knows more about anatomy, physiology, biochemistry, cytology, endocrinology, pathology, and neurology than all the greatest scientists will probably ever know. Your body knows the secret on mind-body-spirit connections and quantum healing. During the years that scientists have been working in their laboratories, attempting to create cells from scratch, your body has been intuitively, easily and silently creating whole networks of cells, tissues, and organs, that function synergistically.

All of this from one microscopic speck! This all happens at immense speed. In fact your body is capable of organizing, both the individual and shared function of around 70 quadrillion cells, which is mind blowing. Your body knows how to cure everything from a tickly cough to something as serious as cancer, and it has already done this innumerable times.

From the very moment that any damage happens to the tissues of your body, your body's intelligence immediately sets to work, organising the healing actions, in the same way a conductor organises an orchestra. Just as the instruments make beautiful music when played at the right time and place within a musical score, your body creates a symphony all of its own.

Messages generated in your brain are sent along nerve channels to every part of your body. The blood vessels near the injury will alter their bioelectrical field to allow white blood cells through the vessel. These white blood cells are the army that march to the site of the wound and begin the healing. At the same time a wall of healing, isolates the damage to a limited area, protecting the rest of the body from further infection.

Microscopic threads of fiber, magically form across the wound and are actually pulled together, to close it. This whole process is happening throughout your body every single minute of every single day. That's because our cells die quite naturally and new cells replace them.

The good news is that we can heal ourselves because the body does have a mind of its own. People from around the world, from different cultures have many names for this "mind". Some people call it the body's wisdom; "inner intelligence". No matter what it is called; our bodies have a wisdom that is nothing short of incredible. When we live with this wisdom, have respect for it, and defer to it, we essentially tap into a source of healing, guidance, and personal power which we cannot bottle.

Candace Pert conducted research and experiments on our cells. Through these experiments it was proved that our cells could survive without their nucleus for between 2 to 4 months. (Pert 1986) This nucleus contains the genes. When cells being experimented on have the genome removed, what is it that controls them, enabling them to survive? Once this genome was removed, the cells continued to search out nutrients from the environment, they continued digesting, excreting and moving around. Without their genetic imprint, was it a powerful type of memory that enabled this to happen?

Candace Pert in 1997 wrote her book Molecules of Emotion. She discovered that neural receptors existed in all cells of the body. Our 'mind' is not just in our head, it is distributed from signal molecules to the whole of our body. She discovered that our emotions not only came through from our environmental information, but the mind can use the brain to 'generate' molecules of emotion and bypass the system. We do this through self-consciousness. What this means is; when we use our consciousness properly, we can bring health to an ailing body. However, inappropriate unconscious control of emotions can just as easily turn a healthy body into an unhealthy one.

Two decades before Candace Perts' work. Robert Ader coined the term Psychoneuroimmunology, or (PNI) for short. This is not a therapy in itself, but merely the name of the science. Dr. Ader believed that there was a definite link between what we think, and our ability to heal and become healthy. This of course is not new. Other cultures for centuries have been saying this, and have in the main, treated patients holistically. They do not separate the mind from the body. We in the West have taken some time to really catch on to the phenomena and we still do not fully integrate this knowledge and understanding into our health care.

Research has continued in looking at the link between the mind and the body, and it has not always been popular with those of the old ideas of health and illness. Psychoneuroimmunology, is based in the main on the central nervous systems, the neuroendocrine system and the immune system and how they inter-relate. The central nervous system is a mass of connections running throughout the body. It allows the brain to send information throughout the body via chemicals. These chemical messengers, are called Neuropeptides, they were once thought to be found only in the brain.

Further research by Candice Pert showed that these neuropeptides are also present in the immune system. These information substances not only affect our physical body but also our emotions as well.

These cells of the body have their receptors on their surface that accepts information coming from the brain. Candace Pert believes that peptides probably provide solutions to every medical problem. These messengers journey through the body, providing vital information and feedback.

Think about a time you saw something that was unpleasant; it's possible you found yourself shivering and then trying to shake off the feeling this event gave you. This shows how fast the information can be transmitted from your thought to your physical body. We create the emotion with input from our brain. It is the limbic system that deals with emotional issues, mainly the hypothalamus.

When Candice Pert, discovered that neuropeptides and neurotransmitters are on the cell walls of the immune system, it showed a close link between emotions and health. Our bodies are in a constant state of adjustment to maintain balance or homeostasis. This balance is maintained as long as the immune system is working at its optimum capacity. The immune system is like your own personal army of defenders on patrol throughout your body, with its own highly complex surveillance system.

The white blood cells are the keys to the immune system; they attack the enemy, suppress them and take over. When our emotions are not expressed in healthy ways, the body will respond by releasing the stress hormones, and weakening our immune systems making us more susceptible to disease.

We can no longer deny the inextricable link between this thought energy, our emotions, including stress, good and bad, and the systems that regulate our bodies. It is therefore very important to express our emotions both verbally and physically in appropriate ways, and look at how our beliefs and thoughts effect our healing.

3. Our Powerful Belief System

Placebo = Belief

To illustrate this thought or mind energy in action; here is the amazing story of a young doctor in the USA way back in 1952. Dr. Mason began treating a 15 year old boy after having him referred from his consultant surgeon. He was not aware at the time that this young boy had a fatal incurable genetic condition.

Dr. Mason believed the boy had been referred because of a severe case of warts, as he had been treating patients with warts using hypnotic suggestion for some time, with much success. When examining the boy he could see 'warts' that covered the whole body apart from a rather small area of healthy skin on the boy's chest. Dr. Mason treated the boy in the same way he treated his other patients with warts, and gave him a session of hypnosis, he asked the boy to use his focus of attention along with the suggestions he had given him, on his arm. The routine was to be followed at least once daily, until his next appointment.

When the boy returned a week later, following the self-hypnotic process that the Doctor had shown him, he found that the boy's arm had begun to heal and the skin was now pink and healthy. The Doctor took his patient to meet with the surgeon who had referred him, who was totally amazed at the outcome.

Once the boy had left the surgery the surgeon explained to Dr. Mason that the condition the boy suffered from was not warts at all, but congenital ichthyosis; a lethal genetic disease that no one before him had ever been able to cure. Despite this revelation, Dr. Mason continued his treatment and the boy made a complete recovery, and went on to lead a long, full and healthy life.

Simply by using the power of hypnosis and his own belief that the treatment would work, both the patient and the Doctor harnessed the thought and mind energy, the patient was able to override his genetic programming. So what was happening with this interaction between the young doctor and the patient? It seems that the determining factor in the positive result of the treatment was belief. Both the doctor's belief in his approach and the patient's belief in what the Doctor would do for him.

The Placebo effect is one area that proves beyond doubt that what we believe has an effect on our physical body. Pain is one of those experiences where our belief about it will affect its severity and its longevity. Belief creates expectation. One of the things in life that creates feelings of happiness or despondency is our expectations. We are always looking to the future. Everything we do on a daily basis is about creating or wanting a better future. So what we think or worry about, more often than not turns into a self-fulfilling prophecy. When we worry, become frustrated, or anxious, or fearful, our body will have a physical reaction to these thoughts. It is this Mind-Body connection that we can use to help relieve the chronic pain that you experience, and provide you with relief and comfort.

The effect of Placebos is a remarkable phenomenon that has been studied extensively for many years. Let me take you back to 1952 and Dr. Mason. This was a perfect example of placebo effect in action. Both the G.P. and the patient believed without question that the condition could be, in fact would be cured. The G.P's belief was strong, the boy's also. This was due to picking up on the G.P's perceptions and accepting them as 'truth'.

What the doctor told the boy, resonated with him. Due to his immense belief, the body healed itself from this condition. This was not a simple case of positive thinking; it was something else, something more profound and unflinching. It consisted of total faith and belief in the process. Their combined perceptions had a positive effect on his body.

As you can imagine, when this result was made public, the doctor was flooded with requests from other patients who suffered with the same condition. The doctor used the same process on numerous patients, but hypnosis proved not to be the cure for this condition that many needed. So what conclusion did the doctor come to?

He believed that the reason for his success was his use of hypnosis combined with his belief in the treatment he gave. Once he was told what the condition was that he was treating, he then had the knowledge of the mass consciousness of the other medical professionals at the time, that the condition was 'incurable'. He too, took on the belief and the opinion, despite his previous success with the 15yr old boy, and despite his upbeat attitude about the outcome with successive patients with the condition.

But how did it work before? The boy was a living breathing example of its success. It was a definite case of mind over matter, and therefore if it can happen once, it can happen again, and it has been proved many times since.

When helping yourself to alleviate the pain you experience, you can now fully embrace this effect, with the immense power of your own internal resources. When you begin to use your own internal power you have at your disposal, an effective efficient tool, free of any side effects, which is capable of treating the dysfunction within your body. There are forces within us that control the molecules that make up our physical body. Quantum physics and quantum mechanics are helping us get closer to how the biology of our body is controlled and regulated, and the mind plays a huge part in this.

Belief in something will produce the positive outcome or the placebo effect. This is where we believe in the drug or treatment and our body becomes well. It is not only used with the administering of drugs, but it has also been tested with surgery. Dr. Moseley, an American surgeon, wanted to test which part of the surgery was having the most positive effect on his patients, so in 2002 he conducted knee surgery on 3 groups of patients. He carried out standard treatment on 2 groups. The surgery was pretty standard practice for varying types of knee problems. One involved flushing the knee, one involved flushing the knee and removing tissue, and the final group had fake surgery. The surgeon opened up the knee and then proceeded stitching it back together.

What was so amazing from this was that the 'fake' surgery patients recovered just as much as the other two groups! It was two years before the patients were told they had fake surgery. This shows that you can achieve miraculous results, when you put your mind to it! These patients believed they had genuinely had an operation and became well and healthy.

This process is being offered by hypnotherapists for weight-loss, using the hypnotic gastric band technique. Many people have had fabulous weight loss from this very technique. Many therapists use hypnosis for the relief of pain during childbirth, and many mothers give wonderful accounts of their calm and pain free birthing of their children.

The point is that all the patients involved in these trials, and the hundreds of others with the same kind of result, all had high expectations of a powerful cure for the pain they experienced, they all got exactly what they expected. Belief creates an expectation.

As with any positive effects from our beliefs, there are also the negative effects, and what is also often termed the Self-fulfilling prophecy. This is known as the 'Nocebo Effect'. It is extremely important to be aware of this whenever you encounter Medical Professionals.

We are bombarded with a massive amount of subliminal messages on a daily basis and patients will observe the medical professionals facial expressions, their words, tone and pitch, their overall body language, all of which, often remove hope in their messages. Telling a pregnant woman that child birth is the worst pain in the world is virtually going to guarantee that she has a painful birth.

Likewise telling someone they only have 3 months to live, will likely mean that person will not be around for very long, if they chose to believe it. Another powerful example of this 'nocebo effect' comes from 1974, where a patient was suffering from oesophageal cancer. It was considered at this time to be a 100% incurable condition.

Even though the medical team treated him with cancer-fighting drugs, they all 'knew' his cancer to be terminal. That 'collective belief' from the whole medical team may well have contributed to his death a few weeks after his diagnosis, as the autopsy showed no cancer in his oesophagus.

There was very little cancer in his body at the time of death, and there was certainly not enough to kill him. The drugs used to treat him had clearly worked to some extent as if there was no cancer at all in his oesophagus!

Some small spots were found in his liver and one small spot in his lung. The patient did die with cancer in his body but he didn't die 'from' cancer. Did he die because he believed he would? Did he pick up on the medical teams' negative outlook? These are the possible effects on a patient when we remove 'hope'. We can all remove hope; Doctors, Teachers, Parents. They, and indeed ourselves, can program us into a belief that we are powerless.

We are not powerless; we can go against the mass consciousness and tread our own path with the use of our own mind power and our own belief. Our belief will colour the world we live in, and your physical body adapts to fit those beliefs.

Many of us have blind faith in God, yet we have not seen God, we have not touched God, we have not had a two-way conversation with God. Yet that unflinching belief affects the way we live our lives. We grew up being educated from a religious or spiritual perspective; we took this on board as 'fact'. Our belief affects everything we do or do not do.

Remember I talked earlier of brainwave patterns and how we can be hypnotised more easily when brainwaves are at Alpha or Theta levels? When we are in a hospital environment, we are extremely focused, we are 'open and receptive' to what the medical professionals tell us, we pick up on the verbal messages, but we also pick up on the subtlety of body language and tonality. Our belief is heightened, and we are in effect in the Alpha state, we are hypnotised by the experience and what we are being told.

"If you believe you can or believe you can't,
You will be right" **(Henry Ford)**

Your beliefs will colour how you see the world. We then physically and mentally adapt to these beliefs. When you fully realise that your beliefs are that powerful, you can see how you can unlock from the prison that your mind and body can become. You can choose what you see. If you choose to see health and relief from pain, your body will respond by growing in health. When you choose to live in fear and doubt, your health will be compromised. You can be shown how to alter your perceptions of your life and your environment. You are not a slave to your genetics; you are master over your own body.

When you learn how to develop mastery over your beliefs, you free yourself from the prison of negative responses, to such an extent that genetic conditions such as the one Dr. Mason faced, can be overcome. Many medics would say that this was simply an anomaly, but there have been numerous cases such as the one I have illustrated, and other research into genetics have shown there are other forces at play, which helps us to question the Medical model of care and how we approach disease, sickness and pain in our society.

It will take some years yet, maybe never, before the Medical Profession and the Pharmaceutical companies acknowledge openly, the power of our minds to heal our bodies. There are the financial implications to why this is, as well as insistent and unequivocal thinking, along with the old suspicion of what hypnosis can do in the hands of someone with dubious intentions.

The multi-million pound drug industry has even harnessed the 'belief effect' when advertising and marketing their products, while at the same time doing their utmost to ridicule the idea when talking of placebo drugs. They tout the miraculous effectiveness of their drugs constantly in the press, and lo and behold, the reported effectiveness went up. It seems that, if you tell someone something often enough, then the belief is installed. Belief is quite clearly catching.

All of this information is to help you to understand the immense power of your own belief system and provide you with evidence of that mind-energy in action. So that you too can harness your powerful belief system, to help you to overcome many health issues. Another report from the USA in 2002 highlighted that; 'in more than half of the clinical trials for antidepressant use, the drugs did not outperform placebo, sugar pills'. (Kirsch et al 2002)

One particular patient found out she had been taking a placebo 'antidepressant' drug back in 1997. She refused to believe this at first because the effects on her were staggering, in that not only had her depression been cured but further brain scans showed that pre-frontal cortex of her brain had been enhanced.

This is the part of the brain that sits in the very front of the brain, just behind your forehead. It controls abstract thinking and thought analysis, it is also responsible for regulating our behavior. This includes mediating conflicting thoughts, making choices between right and wrong, and predicting the probable outcomes of actions or events. It also regulates our thought in terms of both short-term and long-term decision-making. It allows us to plan ahead and create strategies, and also to adjust our actions and reactions in changing situations. Added to this, it helps to focus thoughts, which enables us to pay attention, to learn, and to concentrate. You can see now that someone with depression may have lower functioning in this area of the brain.

Further brain scans following her treatment showed that not only did the patient recover from depression that had been a huge part of her life, but her brain also showed definite improvement in its functioning, which shows us that, the improvements were not made up or 'all in her head'.

The patient also reported that she had side effects, one of which was nausea, from the placebo pills that are a recognised side effect of the drug she thought she was taking! From the small body of evidence that I have room for in this book, I would like you to now consider how your belief system has been affecting your own health and any pain you may be experiencing.

You really can heal yourself and you can, and many people do, create more pain and illness within their body purely due to their belief and their own negative thinking. Could this be you? Just think about it for a few minutes. If patients can recover from genetic conditions, depression, and even have fake surgery, what is the effect on negative thinking in your life?

If you have the power to create pain, illness, and discomfort through your negative thinking and belief, then you also have the power to create health, comfort and wellness in your body too. Isn't that what you want? That is a profound realisation, and one in which I want you to begin to believe you are capable of. It is a switch in mindset, just like flicking the switch to turn on or off your computer or TV.

You can learn how to do this. Your subconscious mind is the part of your mind that is programmed. Think back to when you learned to drive. If you don't drive, then think of something else you were taught how to do. If you were taught well, by a supremely technical instructor, then your driving, or your behaviour will reflect that learning, that programming. In the same way, you learned your beliefs from observing your parents, carers, and teachers, when you were a child. If you remember from the last chapter, I told you that children operate in Alpha and Theta brainwaves, which are the brainwaves of hypnosis. You didn't need to be told anything by your parents or care givers, you simply observed their behaviour. You also downloaded beliefs about yourself, about how the world works, about what is acceptable, unacceptable and about what is possible or not possible.

These beliefs become your 'internal voice' they influence your body and its cellular structure. They do colour your world and give you your perspective. You can change your perspective; you can choose what you believe. If you live with fear, be they personal fears about your health, or some other fear, then you will find yourself living in that world more often than not. However, if you choose to believe in a world of possibilities then your body will respond to that, and grow in health and vitality.

Imagine your world to be one of positive outcomes, of abundance in health, feeling amazingly vital and energized. Doing this imagining on a regular basis and believing in the power of your internal resources, you can begin to feel a rising expectation of the outcome you are looking to create.

Expectation builds more expectation, in an ever-growing cycle of freedom from your previous negative thoughts and the automatic physical responses. You will enjoy the benefits of your changed perspective when you begin to practice the strategies and techniques that involve very little physical effort on your part. Growing in confidence knowing you are now, more in control of your body than you ever believed was possible. There really is no need to live a life of suffering any longer than you have to.

4. The Power of Expectation

Fear

Pain is a complex mix of physical sensations, beliefs and emotional responses. We could say that the basis of physical pain is actually another word, FEAR. A useful acronym that you may be familiar with is: False Evidence Appearing Real.

We were born with only two real fears. Loud noises and fear of falling. So this means that every other fear we have, is created by ourselves, through life experiences as we have grown up. This is neither good nor bad in itself. Sometimes fear can be a life saver. A young child who touches something hot will have an automatic response that teaches the child to stay away from intense heat in the future. The problems begin, when fear goes beyond this initial useful function.

Pain can be made worse by what we think and fear is happening or is going to happen. We fear what may happen to us, we fear what our future holds, we fear the pain will go on forever, we fear the loss of life and opportunities to enjoy life. All this only works to make the pain sensations worse and create a cycle of more negative thinking and pain sensations. This fear can create intense physical sensations.

Let me give you an example of this from the British Medical Journal in 1995: A builder aged 29 came to the accident and emergency department in a hospital in Leicester having jumped down on to a 15 cm nail. It appeared that even the smallest movement of the nail was excruciatingly painful; the patient was sedated with fentanyl and midazolam. Once sedated, the procedure to remove the nail began before taking off the man's boot. The nail was pulled out from below, when his boot was removed, there was a surprise in store for both the doctor and the patient. Despite the nail entering directly through the steel toecap, it had penetrated the boot and went between the toes, meaning his foot was entirely uninjured.

The actual fear of the injury had caused this chap immense pain and yet there was no injury at all! This is the power of expectation. This is something that happens more often than anyone realises. The sensations of fear can be a translation of pain into a physical form. His pain was a 'nocebo' effect (giving a negative outcome) rather than the 'placebo' effect which gives a positive outcome, both based on a person's belief, or in his case 'fear'.

One of the best ways to experience less pain is to reduce fear and anxiety, and increase your confidence, by educating yourself in the many ways you can regain control. Fear and anxiety probably have more power to make pain worse, than any other emotional state, and gaining knowledge and a new perspective are the best treatments you can take.

A confident and happy brain reduces the pain signals more than an anxious one. This has been proven via research in the area of pain, and by clinical observation. When you have an injury or you are told something about your condition, you may expect pain. Along with this expectation you will get an automatic mental image of what you believe is about to happen. The picture in your mind is made up of your current situation, your past experiences and what you believe might happen. Secondly, both the part of your brain that generates the mental picture, and the part that is responsible for registering and processing pain begin to interact. The result is the pain you expected, at a level and intensity that fits your subjective experience and meaning of the pain.

What follows from this are the practical effects; Time off work, social life suffering, relationships suffering, and a never ending cycle of discomfort like a self-fulfilling prophecy of your own making. When people have taken time off work because of pain, the most powerful factor predicting how soon people return to work is whether or not they expect to return to work.

Some health practitioners may have their own perceptions of your recovery based on previous patients they have cared for, and their opinion on your recovery may scare you. It's very important to get as much information as you can possibly find, there is nothing that causes more anxiety than uncertainty. Reduce your fears, by gaining information. These are your real defenses against pain.

As we move through life, every one of us experiences difficulties, we have unexpected situations, there is a gap between what we have now and what we would really like to have. Also when we experience conflict and problems whether they are psychological, emotional, physical or a combination of these, this means there are various parts of the mind that are trying to help us in different ways, but have come into contact with each other. By communicating with the unconscious part of the mind, we can help those parts of the unconscious to come up with a more useful way of working together to create the life of health and happiness that we are looking for.

Another important understanding is that quite often the injury itself and the pain sensations are not in correlation with each other. Yet that is exactly what we all would naturally assume. It is important to remember, that pain is powerfully influenced by perception.

Assumptions

Many of us make assumptions, that a specific injury must produce a specific level of pain. In reality however, this is not necessarily the case, because from evidence produced and events witnessed, there appears to be no correlation between the injury sustained and the level of, type of, and duration of pain that is felt.

Studies have been carried out with those in the military. During warfare, servicemen experience serious, life threatening injuries, including having limbs blown off and yet didn't notice any feelings of pain until after the encounter or battle. Only afterwards when their concentration was brought to the injury, do they then experience the pain sensations. This is due to the shock of the injury and the perceived 'suffering' element we attach to such an injury. Once again an injury in such circumstances may be perceived as 'worse' than it is and the fear kicks in, the pain also kicks in, and only once the wound is cleaned and examined do we find very little to scream about. It also works the other way around too, thankfully, as discussed above.

In the same way, as a far more minor example, how often have you inadvertently cut your finger on paper? You may wince at the thought as you read this, but how often have you done that and not noticed? but as soon as you see it, you immediately feel the pain of that cut.

Pain can also be experienced even after the injury has healed. Residual pain is quite often linked to the 'meaning' of the pain. If we attach a label, such as 'suffering with' then suffer we do. This is a likely cause of the suffering attached to Phantom Limb Pain.

Another effect on our perception of pain is down to our association with previous experiences from within our own family. If there is a medical history of a certain condition, or conditions, such as heart problems within your family for example, and you begin to experience pain in your chest, you are more likely to begin to worry. Once again the fear begins, and you move into the belief it may be the start of heart problems. Once this happens, we then get the never ending internal mind chatter. You begin to constantly look for symptoms, feel pain, you might experience it as severe pain, and it leads you to visit the doctor. However, following a medical from your G.P. you may well be told that all is fine, and then almost as if a miracle happens in the surgery, the pain subsides and often disappears altogether.

This shows how the experience of pain is integrally connected with your own imaginings, or fears, about it. These fears carry that emotional response, that emotional charge, that element of suffering, and the feeling that is attached to the whole experience of pain, and your beliefs about it.

When a person has been living with chronic illness, and thinks that the physical pain associated with it is beyond their control, then what is likely to happen is, they have an emotional experience of feeling helpless, and hopeless against this pain. This leads to other emotional responses such as depression and anxiety, powerlessness, which makes the overall sensation of what they are going through even worse.

The experience of physical pain can also be a manifestation of some emotional feeling or one of a number of unresolved conflicts that are stored at an unconscious level.

This is one of the reasons why hypnotherapists use the subconscious mind to help people unravel any conflicts within themselves. Hypnotherapists can then help people to create the future they really want, free from pain. In the same way we imagine a future we don't want, we can be shown to imagine the future we do want.

In order to make that future life a reality, you have to create a powerful representation of what it's going to be like. Really focus on that future; see it, hear it, feel it, how will your daily life be different, what things will you achieve, that you have put on hold during those health problems? Another significant question is also; What will you have to give up or lose, once you achieve bodily health and wellbeing? What habits of thought and action associated with ill health will have to be left back in the past?

You may have heard the saying 'Be careful what you wish for, you might just get it'! Of course you want health, so allow yourself to be aware that you are going to have to act differently, think differently, and making some real changes in your daily life.

Change

As you change your role in life from being a dependent patient, to being a healthy human being once again, you may well find that your relationships with people close to you will undergo significant changes. Life may be less predictable, which brings its own fears and stresses, but your opportunities will multiply. What this means, is that this whole process does not exist in isolation from the rest of your life.

People in happy relationships appear to suffer less pain and less severe pain than those in unhealthy relationships. Several studies show that people who have a rocky marriage or relationship are likely to experience anxiety and stress and increased risk of health problems. Researchers at University College London tracked about 9,000 people for 12 years and found that negative relationships increase the risk of heart problems by 34 percent. According to researcher John Gottman; an unhappy marriage can increase the chances of illness by 35 percent.

A happy marriage or long term live-in relationship helps ease the agony of arthritis, research suggests. The findings, published in the Journal of Pain, support earlier studies which found the crippling disease progressed more slowly in happily married than single people.

Rheumatoid arthritis patients who had the support of a loving spouse or partner, reported less joint pain and better mobility than those who were single or whose marriage was on the rocks. Scientists believe the emotional stability that a strong marriage/relationship provides, also has a powerful effect on physical sensations, such as pain.

Now that you're committed to achieving the best for your body, think about other ways you can move away from your previous experience of pain, towards a comfortable and healthy future. Think about what you eat. Your body needs predominantly water-rich foods, fresh fruit and vegetables, salads, and water itself. Making these foods the centre of your diet will give you the resources it needs to rebuild itself in a healthy strong way.

Consider doing some simple light exercise and movement, such as Tai Chi or swimming. Many of the physical pains in the head neck and shoulders, also in the back are often due to the misuse of our body, sitting at a desk all day, slouching on the sofa, our bodies are not designed for such inactivity long term. Getting up often, stretching out the muscles, loosening them up, will all help to ease tensions, stiffness and the pain in those areas.

Another thing to be aware of is; when you begin to become actively involved in an activity or involved with other people, you become so absorbed with it that the pain is simply forgotten in all but extreme cases. If you have been in pain for some time, can you remember getting together with family or friends on a public holiday for instance, where there were times during that day, you forgot about the pain entirely? Becoming involved in new things, new hobbies etc. can act as the perfect distraction. Perhaps, visiting tourist attractions in your area, becoming involved in community activity or taking up a hobby or interest that has fallen by the wayside, anything in fact that you positively enjoy doing.

Don't have the energy or motivation? Well think how can I find that energy? that motivation?

You will find answers coming to you that will help you to find it. The point is, that finding time to do new and different things; your experience of life will be different. Your senses are filled with new and inspiring things and these new activities can lead to the mobilisation of those inner resources that will create your future life of bodily comfort.

When we first become aware of pain in our body, our first response is to take painkilling drugs. We then attempt to distract ourselves from it. When the pain continues and it becomes Chronic Pain, there is a tendency to begin to harden against it and fight it. The problem with this is that by trying to evade our suffering, we create more of it in the form of secondary suffering.

5. Thoughts and Emotions

We now have an understanding of how our beliefs, thoughts and emotions can add to our pain experience. When we add the suffering element, then it can be very difficult to get out of that negative cycle of thinking. This emotional element of suffering, is itself made up of two parts, the immediate physical pain we are experiencing (primary suffering), and our memory of past experiences of pain, and our anticipation of more pain in the future (secondary suffering). (Birch 2008) It gets to the point that when we experience any feeling coming from the affected part of the body, our automatic response is to classify it as pain.

Your primary suffering is the immediate physical discomfort that you would experience as a result of the illness, or injury you have. It is safe to say that we are unlikely to be able to do anything about this acute pain and the Primary suffering, other than to accept it as part of the illness or injury. We stub our toe, and we accept it's going to hurt as the brain registers the pain. Once the brain understands that the injury is not life threatening, then the level of pain or discomfort begins to lessen as our brain disregards the sensations.

The secondary suffering is the emotional part that we all have when we react to the primary suffering. When pain and discomfort become Chronic (long term) we may well experience feelings of anger. We can be fearful; we may become depressed, anxious and feel hopeless about the future. We begin projecting a whole host of negative outcomes, negative possibilities that we do not want. It's that instinctive response to any unpleasant situation that creates more of what we do not want.

We then find ourselves going in ever-decreasing circles of despair, and when this happens we tense our body, we hold our breath and grit our teeth. The old 'stiff upper lip' of grin and bear it. However, what this does is make the pain far worse, because as we all know, tension in our body creates more pain and discomfort. Relaxation eases and smoothes out tension, helping us to feel far more comfortable, and the pain then starts to become manageable.

Learning to become more aware of our body tensing and resisting, helps us to do something about it, before it gets out of hand or feel overwhelming. We can learn new and more powerful ways to reduce the experience of secondary suffering. What then happens is you massively improve your quality of life, whether or not the cause of the primary suffering worsens, as it may do, depending on the reasons for it.

PRIMARY SUFFERING
CHRONIC PAIN AND ILLNESS
(in the case of basic unpleasant sensations)

LEADING TO

RESISTANCE

AND

SECONDARY SUFFERING

(thoughts and emotions)

In other cases, there can be some deep seated emotions at a subconscious level, which have been left unattended and not worked through, and which may well take the form of a physical pain, usually this happens without any physical reason. In situations such as this, the pain is in effect a substitute for the expression of some emotion or other.

When we have negative thoughts they can very quickly begin to take over, and it's as if we are running a horror movie inside our heads, and like a snowball rolling down a hill, it picks up speed and grows to immense proportions. Of course we can have the same effect with positive thoughts and emotions, finding that they grow and blossom into something wonderful.

Whenever we have a situation or a change happening in our lives, we tend to jump into the future in our thoughts and we can imagine all kinds of negative consequences, even if the change is something we want and look forward to, and we are always more inclined to think about the negative consequences rather than the positive ones.

If you experience chronic pain, then the thought conversation you have with yourself can go something like this; "Oh no! This pain is awful in my back, I can't cope with this all day today" 'I really can't go on like this; is this my future, day in and day out for the rest of my life?' These thoughts will then generate an emotional component; you feel desperate, overwhelmed, out of control, powerless, become anxious, frustrated, sad. You might decide to go to bed and sleep as it's the only relief you get. Maybe you can take stronger medication. This may make you drowsy and you fall asleep that way.

What is actually happening here is; the experience of pain is not only due to the injury, it's also due to what you have been telling yourself in that internal conversation. It's about the 'meaning' you have put on to the pain sensations, 'awful' 'can't cope' 'hopeless' 'powerless'. You have taken on the role of victim to the pain. If you take a different approach, the pain becomes manageable, and you become more the driver rather than the passenger. Like this: "Oh oh, there's that pain, ok, just breathe, I know it's going to hurt for a while but it will pass soon, all I have to do is to relax into this and breathe through it. Focus on something else for a while, my medication isn't due just yet, and I can manage this until then'. This way of thinking is a much more helpful way, and more realistic way to manage the pain sensations when they happen, even if the pain is intense.

What you are doing in this second example is changing your focus, from how awful the pain is, to what you can do to cope and manage it. Your negative thoughts about pain have an impact on how you view the pain sensations. How you feel emotionally, and what you feel you are able to do when in pain. Added to this, you are more likely to feel the full force of your emotional distress, which leads to more muscle tension, making that pain far worse.

You also generate that hyper-aroused state in your nervous system, causing more pain messages in your body, adding more pain into the mix. Negative thoughts and emotions also cause us to have self-defeating behaviours. This can mean being less active, isolating ourselves and refusing to mix socially, and relying too much on the prescribed medication, which can also affect our pain with the added side effects that often come with them.

Quite often the thoughts and images we have about the pain we experience, and life events in the moment, are related to those deeper beliefs. You may be one of those people who have chronic pain and believe that the pain has taken over your life. You may believe that the pain makes you a weak person, or inadequate in some way. You may believe that your body is broken.

There may be beliefs about the relationships with your GP or medical staff; that they don't care, that others don't understand what you are going through, and lastly you may well have those self-defeating beliefs about your future, feeling destined to be in pain forever.

Positive Thinking

This is not another book on the power of positive thinking. On the contrary, positive thinking is not enough. It takes more than thinking positive to create the changes in your body that will help you alter your perception of pain. It is true that when we focus on the things we want to happen, then we are more likely to achieve that result. After all it's true you always get more of what you focus on. However, we need a combined effort of eliminating the negative and accentuating the positives, to re-direct our thoughts and our mind-energy in this way. From the evidence in this book, you may now have a deeper understanding of the conscious mind and the subconscious mind, and how they are interconnected and interdependent.

It is our conscious mind (the creative part) that brings forward the positive thoughts. Our subconscious mind is the 'habit' part. It works from a much deeper level; it uses our instincts as well as the learned responses we have picked up over our lifetime. They come from all the situations and events we have either witnessed or been a part of. We then, with the help of the subconscious, replay these behaviours and responses over and over again, creating the habitual behaviours and thought patterns we often feel unable to change.

Your subconscious mind is a million times more powerful than the conscious mind; Processing 20,000,000 bits of information or stimuli from our environment, as opposed to the 40 bits that our conscious mind interprets. Not only this; but the subconscious constantly monitors both your external and internal environments, triggering almost instantaneous responses without you being consciously aware of them.

You can now see that due to the immense amount of information coming in, being held, and being processed, your subconscious mind is the 'powerhouse' of your brain. This will give you some idea of which part of your mind will win when your conscious wishes come into conflict with your subconscious programming.

For instance, you may repetitively say positive affirmations to yourself that you are worthy or that your body will heal, but what if you were told something different over and over as a child? What if you picked up the subtle body language and behaviours of others repeatedly, that contradict the affirmation? What if you believe that you were not, or are not loveable, or you picked up the message somewhere that you are worthless, and you then went on to believe that? Any affirmations are going to fall short of the outcome you want.

What do you think might be the outcome if you were told 'you were always a sickly child'? All of your conscious efforts at affirmations designed to change your life, will be negated. So, you may well ask how all this goes towards helping you use your mind to relieve your pain?

Due to extensive research and using the information gained from it, therapists and pain specialists now have a deeper understanding of what contributes to the pain experience. Hypnosis and meditation are two powerful ways to help people manage pain and discomfort and promote healing. These methods have always been used to create a relaxed state of mind and body, which as you now know, help to create comfort and a sense of wellbeing.

Along with this, Cognitive Behavioural strategies go a long way in helping people have a more realistic view. Cognitive Behavioural Therapy or (CBT) was first used to treat depression, and is an extremely useful strategy for this. It also helps people to identify the emotions, thoughts, and behaviours that might have a negative impact on pain. Along with the other influences such as family situations, social situations, culture and any physical disability that is present.

Hypnosis, meditation and cognitive behavioural strategies teach you how to reduce pain, how to be less affected by it, and enhance your daily life experience by bringing you more in control and feeling less like a victim.

Being a victim of pain does appear to have some perceived 'benefits' for some people. These perceived benefits are often subconscious and hidden from the person with pain, and rarely acknowledged. Unlike hidden agenda which is only hidden from others, and the person with pain may well be aware of them and operate from them, again it is rarely acknowledged.

Holding on to pain

This may indeed sound like an incredible statement. Why, you may ask would anyone wish to experience pain and hold onto it? What is there to gain from having pain on a daily basis? There are several possible reasons for this. People who experience pain are also experiencing a level of care, attention and love which they may believe will be difficult to obtain if they recovered their health and wellness. Also in some cases, there can be financial and material gain, which actually serves to prolong it.

Compensation payments for work related injuries, can act as an incentive for pain to continue. No one but the person will know what their reasons are, possibly not even the person themselves. The pain can be a 'get out of jail card' in the monopoly game of life, where they are free from responsibilities that they find difficult. None of this suggests that the pain is invented or imaginary. On the contrary, pain is always real to the person experiencing it.

Freud used the phrase 'secondary gain' to explain the phenomena when treating phobia. He noticed that some people prefer to keep their phobia because it serves a hidden purpose "the motive for the illness, the advantage gained from having it. It was also noted that the patient can be quite disappointed if the therapist succeeds in helping them to get rid of it. Secondary gain is the positive practical advantages gained by using the negative symptoms, in this case, Pain, to influence or manipulate." (Dr Patrick Jemmer, Northumbria University Newcastle UK)

For some people pain, becomes their identity. They may have lived with the pain for such a long time that they may believe they would not know how to 'be' any other way. We human beings want to fit in and stand out, there are quite often times when someone might not know how else to achieve this. A disability is not very good for you to fit into society, but it does very well at letting you stand out.

As a result, disability can become an identity. It may not be an identity we want. We might prefer that we were a wealthy Executive Officer of a huge company, but what if you believe you cannot create that identity, or the one you want? When we come across something that distinguishes us from the rest of the crowd, we tend to stick with it; Holding on, even if it is pain.

An elderly client of mine had been experiencing severe shoulder pain for some years. Even though she had contacted her GP and undergone all possible investigations, medications, physiotherapy, heat treatments, and was recovering from recent exploratory surgery, the consultant had told her "there is nothing physically wrong with your shoulder." In spite of this, the pain was still present and real to her. After going through the usual sessions of my Pain Control Programme, and only getting the minimum result expected, I felt I had to ask a question that had been coming up for me. I asked her *"What benefits are you getting from the pain and how has your life changed since the pain began?"*

This lady struggled to find any benefit at first, but following further discussion, she did say that her husband now helps with the house-work and garden, which he had never ever done before. Her son, who lived close by but had rarely visited before, had become a regular visitor, taking her shopping in the car and doing the DIY. She also said that her daughter would now find other babysitters, rather than bringing the children to be looked after three times a week.

Yet another client had experienced a severe injury from a car accident 6 years earlier. At the time he was working in an extremely stressful environment as the manager of a team in a call centre. The client had recovered fully from the injury, and yet the pain was so intense he had remained on leave from work the whole time. Once again careful questioning revealed the secondary gain, that while he was 'ill' he didn't have to return to the stressful job that he basically hated, and he also received the other perceived benefits we spoke of earlier.

These are just a couple of the many examples from my own clients, of why we hold on to pain. This doesn't mean that we intend to hold on to pain, it just highlights that many people do indeed hold on, and once they are open to looking at their situation, they do admit to having clung to it more than they realized. The result of this was that they only served to prolong the misery and hold themselves back. If this sounds familiar, please be hopeful. Typically in the face of pain, we believe that all we can do is passively wait. But if we are holding on to pain in any way, we can at least get rid of some of it.

Caroline Myss talks of 'woundology'.(1997) She says that many people use their pain, be it physical, mental or emotional, as a kind of currency. We socialise, and interact with others, who are in similar situations to us. She also controversially says; it's also a very subtle type of manipulation or control, in a socially acceptable way. We may ask someone what they are going to do now that they are looking better, or when they are going back to work.

The person answers this by going straight to their 'wound'. "Oh I can't do anything now I have had such a hard time, and I'm in such pain, I CAN''T do anything".

The next thing that happens is we, the questioner, have no other option other than to back off. We don't challenge this, and instead we sympathise with platitudes and give that 'poor you' expression on our faces.   The person holding on to the pain may believe there are benefits to holding on, or they may not even know they are doing this.

Using our wounds or our pain carries a high price. It's the price we pay for communicating via our pain. We appear to be having a simple conversation; we do it to get to know someone new. How often have you entered a conversation with someone, and before you even know it, you have their history, bad illnesses, horrendous relationships and other losses? You can then identify with them by giving your own list in an attempt to empathise.

Woundology, is the way we use our pain to explain why we can't or won't be able to do something. Instead of saying a simple 'no' we go into all the reasons why, it's not possible, using our 'illness' to do so. Challenging someone who does this will mean you are likely to lose a friend, because you no longer play the same game as them.

You don't play by the same rules any longer. You no longer serve their wound. It might be interesting to take a look at how other cultures view pain and how they work with it, rather than fight it, and how different and much more helpful this approach is.

6. Cultural Differences and the Pain Experience

Conditioning

As we evolved as human beings, so did our limbic system. Our brains increased in size, and more and more of our cells developed to respond to ever more varieties of external signals and stimulus from our environment. We were then able to generate reflex responses, based on our instincts, and then we also began to learn from experiences. This is what we call Conditioning. A prime example of this conditioning was discovered by Ivan Pavlov, a Russian physiologist, who discovered classical conditioning by observing his dogs.

Pavlov noticed that his dogs would salivate, whenever he entered the room, even though he was not bringing any food. He then went on to conduct some simple experiments and what he did, was effectively train his dogs to salivate whenever he rang a bell and offered food at the same time. After many times of doing this he would then ring the bell but offer no food. However, by the time he did this, the dogs were so conditioned/programmed to expect the food, that when he rang that bell, it set off their salivate reflex even though no food appeared. This is what we call 'unconscious' learned reflex behaviour.

Another unconscious learned behaviour is when we drive from A to B and we miss part of the journey. You do not need to be consciously active in the process of driving. You know by the sound of the engine when to change up or down the gears. You stop at red lights, slow down for other vehicles. Your subconscious reflexes are in operation. You drive on 'autopilot'.

The subconscious operates by reflexes (without intention) it isn't governed by reason. We are all conditioned by our environments, and our cultural heritage. There are certain behaviours and practices that we engage in that are conditioned into us.

Perceptions

Remember we spoke about perception? Well, our brains' capacity to learn perception means we also take on board other people's perceptions. As you grew up your teachers, parents and other adults all had their own perceptions of how the world worked and they instilled some of these onto you. These perceptions could have been good or bad. They quite often conflict with your own perceptions until you grow and have the ability to go out and prove differently.

Once we take on board someone else's perceptions as being 'true' their perceptions are hardwired into our brain and also become our truth. So if you take on board your G.P's perception that a certain drug will work for the pain you have, it becomes true for you, helping you experience the relief that you are looking for. You are effectively hypnotised into believing in the prescribed cure being offered. Likewise, in other cultural traditions, if they are told by their spiritual leaders, or their local 'medicine man/woman' that something will cure them, then they too, take this on board as being real.

Our problems begin when someone else's perception is wrong. What we have then is akin to a virus being downloaded onto your computer. We have a 'misperception'. We then use these in the same way as before, but with misperception it negatively affects our thoughts, and consequently our behaviours. We get the nocebo effect of which I spoke earlier.

This illustrates how all our responses are controlled by our perceptions and not all of these are real or accurate. Everything you hear is filtered through your perceptions, everything you see is filtered through perceptions, smell, taste and touch are all filtered through our perceptions, and the meaning we give everything.

Not all spiders are poisonous, not all dogs are dangerous. So what we essentially have with perception is a set of beliefs.

This is powerfully significant because it means we are not victims of our genetic makeup or others' beliefs, or our self-sabotaging behaviours, once we learn to harness that powerful subconscious mind.

African and Asian Cultural Perspective

The experience of pain and indeed the lack of it, is also influenced by cultural factors. In the West, we are expected to fight pain, kill pain, conceal pain, or to have the stiff upper lip and bare it bravely. In Southern Europe, it is much more acceptable to express feelings of suffering, probably as a result of these differences, the level of heat from the sun that we might consider too much, when we visit the Mediterranean on our annual holidays, are considered only 'warm' by those who actually live there. In some other cultures, pain can be almost and even completely eliminated.

In certain parts of India, they carry out rituals where a member of their community is chosen to represent the power of their Gods. In what is called a 'Hook hanging ceremony'. During this ceremony he (it's always a 'he') is transported in a cart, to the surrounding villages in his area blessing the new-borns, the children and blessing the crops.

Strong metal meat hooks are attached by ropes to a cart with a cross beamed structure. The chosen one then enters a trance like state, an hypnotic state, and once he indicates he is sufficiently hypnotised, these steel hooks are then pushed under and through his skin and muscles on both sides of his back. I can almost feel you squirming! The cart then begins its journey, travelling from village to village with the man holding onto the ropes. Once he reaches the village, he then swings freely, suspended only by the metal hooks embedded in his back.

Throughout the whole ceremony, there is no evidence to show that he experiences any pain at all. He appears to be in a state of total Euphoria. How can this be? What is going on here?

In East Africa, people still undergo a procedure, known as Trepanning. This procedure is believed to relieve pressure from within the skull and therefore eases pain. Along with this there is also the belief that it releases 'demons' from the person.

Trepanning involves cutting the scalp and underlying muscles to expose the bone of the skull. This is done without the aid of anaesthesia. The skull is then drilled using a Trepanner and throughout the whole procedure, the person is seen looking unconcerned and completely at ease. This level of ease and calmness is largely due to the patients 'trust' in the doctor, along with their high expectation of gaining the relief they are looking for, along with their conditioning, and all the other cultural and psychological factors, it means they experience no discomfort whatsoever.

What the peoples of India and Africa are doing is successfully drawing on their inner subconscious resources, which help them experience their own level of calmness, in situations where we might assume it to be impossible to do. They seem to have an inner awareness of their own power, to close down the pain gates within the spinal cord, focusing on the benefits they are receiving, rather than the pain they are currently experiencing. Is there more going on? Could it be that within these cultures they are much more spiritually aware.

One commonality between all cultures however, is the belief and/or awareness of a deep creative centre in all human beings. A creative centre that is in some way connected to the infinity of the universe and its healing and creative powers.

The various religious and spiritual belief systems on the planet all have in common the role of ritual, no matter how much they differ in other areas. They have mystery, initiation rites, a quest for and achievement of mystical states of being, even those philosophical belief systems that reject the concept of the supernatural, nevertheless find themselves developing secularised rituals.

At some higher order of existence, these features of the human experience tap into something deep inside ourselves. The realm of the spiritual, however we each individually wish to define that word, seems to have a deep and meaningful correspondence within something at the core of ourselves. There must be a part of all human beings that looks to approach an awareness or reality, which goes way beyond the scientific or logical explanation.

An awareness approached through mystical experiences. One thing that connects all of these rituals, trances or other worldly experiences, is their healing transformative powers, and especially with the absence of any pain sensations. We have just discussed the ritual of blessing in India and Africa where the celebrant blesses the crops and children while in an exalted state of awareness in which there are no sensations of pain.

This phenomenon has been witnessed in other religious spiritual and mystical cultures around the globe. In the western world, as early as the 2nd century AD the philosopher Lamblichus wrote about divination in 'De mysteriis'. He said, *"when someone was in a trance, it seemed as if sensation and life has been suspended, he has ceased to feel pain and has not felt the application of fire"*.

Every major religious or spiritual tradition has remarkably similar experiences. We all have our mystics; our gurus, our spiritual leaders, and many have learned how to tap into this power, to move away from daily experiences and awareness, and to enter a state that is fundamentally different. A state that is something way beyond our logical understanding and something we cannot often put into words, where being numb to pain is one powerful feature.

Different cultures follow their own unique paths to achieving a mystical experience. The process of meditation comes from concepts of thought, from India from which Hinduism, Buddhism, Yoga and other related systems practice. It is now widely recognised by the medical profession in the West, to be a wonderful way of helping people who experience long term pain, to manage and control it. The people of Asia and Africa have developed their own concepts and include the belief that there is a vital life energy called 'Prahna' that flows from the universe, and within the human body, it is believed there are 7 Chakras or energy centres, each with its own specific colour through which this 'Prahna' flows.

The word Chakra means wheel, or disc or circle. It is believed that as the prahna flows up through the body, each chakra is then energised and the wheel spins rapidly. They are often compared with flowers which open up like sunflowers when faced with the sun, as the life energy flows upwards through them.

Somewhere deep inside every individual, no matter their religion, culture or background, there lives this ability to tap into this kind of experience. The process has no intention of promoting any religious spiritual or mystical belief. What I am describing, is simply that powerful inner resource of all human beings, no matter where you live on the planet. That resource that we can all be taught to tap into, if and when we need to, in order to help ourselves relieve and control the pain sensations. From the research quoted earlier in this book, it appears that science has begun to actually catch up with, and prove the existence of this 'unseen force' so why not learn how to use it, for your benefit?

When you allow yourself to be open to using this experience, then you have an extraordinarily powerful means of moving towards that bodily comfort that is so important to you. So whatever your religious, spiritual or mystical beliefs are, I invite you to open your mind and body to this experience that holds amazing potential for you.

What I'm attempting to illustrate here, is that pain never only exists as a purely physical sensation in isolation. There is always an emotional element, an emotional connection to it. Whether this be a desirable one e.g. giving birth, or an undesirable one such as the emotional suffering associated with long term chronic pain. It also appears that we have a deeper knowing, directly relating to your inner core of being human. It is this core that we refer to when we experience things that emotionally move us.

When we experience the birth of a child, a sunset or sunrise, or when we hear a particular piece of music or song that can bring us to tears, these things evoke thoughts, and emotions deep within us. Throughout all cultures of the world, music is one of those things that can have a profound effect on our feelings of wellbeing, and resonates to our heart and soul, whether you believe in a soul or not.

7. Music and its effect on the pain experience

Evidence of Healing

When we use Hypnosis and Meditation for any issue, more often than not, music is played during sessions to induce trance and to lull the mind into a relaxed state. Music has been used for centuries in this way for healing purposes. It can be more powerful than words to convey a message, and it has a way of speaking to the emotional centre within each and every one of us. Music has been used for thousands of years to promote relief from pain, be it emotional, spiritual or physical. As far back as the time of the Ancient Greeks, there was a belief that music was important to help heal the mind body and spirit of the patient.

Native Americans used singing and chanting. Sound healing using singing bowls, drumming and other forms of music are used to help balance the bodies systems and strengthen the mind-body connections. It helps relieve stress and this ultimately creates a sense of wellbeing.

There have been studies to show that music can lower blood pressure, heart rate and breathing.

Music plays a powerful role in healing within many cultures of the world, and is still used along with other practices in the absence of powerful painkilling medication. Rhythmic drumming, singing, chanting etc. have a hypnotic effect on patients and altering their state of awareness, which draws on powerful unconscious resources, which help embed the strong suggestion that a remedy is available.

But how is it that music has such a meaningful and therapeutic effect on us? What is it about music that affects us in such powerful ways, and has such a profound effect upon our brains? During the second World War, music began being used to help US veterans overcome shell-shock, as it was noted that they recovered more quickly after listening to the local musicians, some hospitals even began recruiting their own bands, and back in 1944 the very first music therapy degree programme began at Michigan state university. Professional music therapists now work within the health care arena in the US mainly within cancer care.

It is no surprise therefore, that much of the research into how music has powerful positive effects has been in the area of cancer care, to help reduce pain and anxiety. It was even reported by patients themselves that they also had a reduced incidence of nausea which was a common side effect of the chemotherapy treatment. Other research studies proved that music therapy is useful in short term pain, as well as reducing the intensity of pain when it was used with pain killers, improving the level of comfort, relaxation and improved patients' quality of life.

Music seems to speak the language of our primitive brain centres, where our motivation and emotions live. When we hear a piece of music, the cerebellum and amygdala are activated as our brain responds to the beat of the music. It even has the power to conjure up images as well as mood and emotion, which add to the whole experience. It is of course, capable of generating the opposite to relaxation and peace too.

After all, music is basically sound, some sounds can have us wanting to run for the hills to escape, or it can trigger negative emotions and desires, purely by how it is perceived by our brain. Have you ever felt that some sound is an assault on your senses? That is the immense power that sound can have on each of us.

When we mix certain sounds together, and create music with tone, pitch, melody etc. it appears to have an effect on our primitive emotional centres. It really doesn't matter what genre of music it is, as long as you enjoy it, then you will experience the positive effects, as it connects to the pain centres and reduces the level of intensity, due to its relaxing effects.

If you have ever bought an hypnosis or meditation CD, you will find gentle restful music being played in the background of your awareness. Music alone is one of the ways to harmonise your bodies systems. There are certain parts of the brain that can only be accessed through music, and through history in all cultures, music has been used for its healing properties. Music has a wonderful power to draw on the wonderful healing properties of your body and mind.

We all know how owners of supermarkets and shopping malls pipe music throughout their buildings, it's all done in an attempt to lull us into a state where we are more inclined to buy products, and it really works. Our brainwaves rhythm slows to the alpha level, and before you know it, you have almost bought shares in the company, when all you needed was a hair brush! It's specifically designed to alter our mood. Another way that music alters our mood is through the power of film.

When the boy meets girl, boy kisses girl, girl melts into his arms, and the camera pans out and blurs as the passion increases. Or when the hero of the hour is on his way to save the day, and of course we can't forget the horror movie music that sends shivers down your spine and can cause several weeks of sleepless nights.

It is no wonder that the interest in music and its healing power, have grown over the years. How often have you put on some music to cheer yourself up? Or played a song that reminds you of a lost love, so you can wallow in those feelings?

Music does indeed have the power to heal and the power to take us even further down into the pits of despair. When we are sad, depressed and alone, even our voices change. It is one of the first sounds we pick up on when someone close to us is 'not themself'.

Think about the last time someone called you on the phone. Could you tell from their tone and pitch of voice if they were sounding well and happy, or could you discern that something was wrong? Has anyone ever said the same to you? 'You're not sounding like yourself today'? We know that our voice changes depending on the state of our emotional and physical health.

When I was coming out of a period of grief some time ago, many people who knew me told me they knew when I was better on some days, or worse due to how my voice changed. It was music that I used to both remember my loved one and also to forget my pain. It really did bring me out of that difficult place, as the music resonated with something deep inside, and the healing began.

Resonance

The human body has its own rhythm and resonance as we have already touched upon. Various songs & music aligns with this resonance, and that is why we often feel better after listening to certain types of music. From the dawn of time, we have been subjected to the sounds of nature all around us and it appears that we resonate with certain sounds. We then attempted to replicate them in a systematic way, and this is how music began to be formed. The history of music is the history of attempting to synthesize the sounds of nature all around us.

From the day we were conceived, the cells of our body have been subject to sound. The sound of the mother's body, her heart beat, her breathing, and the blood coursing through her veins into the umbilical cord, feeding and nourishing the growing child within. There are a myriad of sounds from her body systems, all being transferred to the cells of the developing foetus.

There have been many studies on the effect of music on the baby while in the womb. Several different genres of music are played to the pregnant mother to register the effect on her baby. The unborn child has been noted to respond in various ways depending on the sound heard.

These sounds resonate with the developing human brain and maybe this could be one of the reasons why music touches us to our very core. Our cells have memory and once the child is born and the music is played again to the child, it responds to the music once again.

This fascinating research adds to the continuing studies of the effects of music on the human brain. When music is played at certain speeds, beats per minute, it appears to have a more calming peaceful effect. One such genre of music that has been studied to have beneficial effects is Baroque music. Its slow tempo at 55-65 beats per minute are in tempo with the hearts' resting rate. This type of music is often used in music therapy with children who have some form of disablement, to help and encourage them to learn and engage.

When the music is played it has been found to lower blood pressure and slow the heartbeat down. Also EEG readings have shown changes to the brainwaves occur, in that the fast beta (everyday waking state) waves that we discussed earlier in this book, gradually decreased by around 6% while the alpha waves (the relaxing waves) rose by 6% it also appeared to synchronise both the left and right hemispheres of the brain, and this means that the brain can be more productive. Learning new skills and making it easier to retain information.

The Bulgarian Psychiatrist, Georgi Lazanoff (2006) showed an increased capacity for learning, by playing Baroque music to his students, and asking them to breathe in rhythm to the beat. You will have experienced the power of sound and music yourself many times I'm sure, maybe when a piece of music or a song brought you to the verge of tears. It's true to say that our health can be strongly affected by music. It's as if the very energy of music, its frequency and vibration touch you in such a way, where nothing else can.

You may be thinking right now "I don't like Baroque music, or I don't like classical music." and that's ok, because all of the beneficial health effects I've mentioned here can be found in any music that resonates with you. There's that word again. It's true that Baroque and New Age music have been reported to be very successful in treating insomnia. Likewise, another study used various genres of music, ranging from pop music, to country, to jazz, classical, heavy metal and rock and roll, all to help ease the pain of childbirth.

The study showed that over half of the birthing mothers who listened to music during the birth of their child, did not require any anesthesia. Music really does have the power to raise the level of endorphins, one of your body's natural pain killers, into your bloodstream.

Everything has resonance because everything has a frequency and a vibration. Every individual molecule vibrates and resonates in some way with the next and the next. The universe we live in is made up of this resonance and vibration.

There are various strands of alternative and complementary medicine that are being used to inform our medical model of health care, and it appears that in some areas, science is beginning to catch up with what ancient healers from other cultures around the world and mystics have known for so long, when it comes to health.

Music does help us to stay in the flow of this healing energy. One of the oldest medical systems in the world is that of Ayurveda, and the use of music helps to replicate the rhythms of the natural world. It is understood that as our body senses these natural energies, our mind is more open to the natural link towards health and wellbeing. Music in the use of hypnosis and meditation to reduce and eliminate pain, can be your new prescription to a pain free future, should you choose.

8. How the Brain registers Pain

The human body is a combination of various systems. We have a circulation system, a respiratory system, cardiovascular system, digestive system, immune system, limbic system, sympathetic nervous system and others.

When scientists wanted to find out how all these systems worked, they had to spend a lot of their time dissecting the organs of the body. By investigating the organs of the body they became more knowledgeable about their structure on a molecular level. It is from these investigations and their findings, that they developed the medical model of care that we are all so familiar with. The 'pill for all ills' approach.

When we experience pain, we automatically reach for painkillers to ease the discomfort that we feel. But how does the brain actually register pain? There are several theories:

Signals from the affected area travel through the central nervous system to the brain, and these are then interpreted as pain. We all know that quite often, that pain can have a useful function. It acts as a warning that a part of our body is in danger, or has been damaged, and this encourages us to take the action necessary to deal with it.

We place a hand on the hot stove; we pull our hand away quickly before any significant damage is done. You twist your ankle; the pain encourages you to rest it, avoid walking on it for a while to help it to heal. You may strap it up to give it extra support and reduce swelling in the area. These are examples of useful pain; it's our early warning signal.

However when it goes beyond this, we then have a problem. Chronic pains; these are typically those that go on longer than 6 months, such as lower back, muscular, nerve damage, phantom limb pain, CFS/ME, Fibromyalgia, various forms of Arthritis and some skin diseases. It's as if that warning light continues flashing long after the problem has been fixed. What about when the problem cannot be fixed, and you are told that pain is the legacy you have inherited with the condition?

How do we account for the fact that pain is such a varied and subjective experience? In that we experience that pain in an individual and unique way.

Pain can persist even after injuries have healed. This is what we usually refer to as chronic pain. Chapman and Bonica (1985) identify three types of chronic pain:

· pain that lasts after the normal feeling of a disease or an injury.

· pain associated with a chronic medical condition, such as a degenerative disease or a neurological condition.

· pain that develops and persists in the absence of identifiable organic problem.

People's experience with chronic pain also depends on two factors:

· whether the underlying condition is benign or is malignant and worsening.

· whether the discomfort exists continuously, or occurs in frequent and intense episodes.

Using these factors, Dennis Turk, Donald Meichenbaum, and Myles Genest (1983) have described three types of chronic pain:

1. Chronic/recurrent pain stems from benign causes, and we can recognise it as repeated and intense episodes of pain, inter-spaced by periods without pain. A couple of examples of chronic/recurrent pain are migraine headaches and tension headaches; another example is myofascial pain; a syndrome that typically involves shooting, or radiating but dull pain in the muscles and connective tissue of the head and neck, and sometimes in the back.

2. Chronic/intractable/benign pain means that a person experiences discomfort that is present all of the time, with various levels of intensity. It is not related to an underlying malignant condition. Chronic low back pain is one such example.

3. Chronic/progressive pain is recognised by continuous discomfort, usually from a malignant condition, such as cancer, and becomes increasingly intense as the underlying condition worsens. One such condition that frequently produces chronic/progressive pain is rheumatoid arthritis.

Theories of Pain

Specificity Theory

During the 1600 century, the French philosopher Rene Descartes suggested that the intensity of pain was related to the level of injury. In effect, you could stub your toe and it would give you minimal pain, but if you broke your toe then this would cause more injury and therefore more pain. It is still generally accurate when we are talking about certain type of pain such as 'acute pain' but it doesn't answer the questions provoked from those who experience chronic pain, where there is no obvious physical or mechanical injury in our body.

Later Von Frey (1895) also followed with the theory that the body has a separate sensory system for perceiving pain, and this system has its own special 'receptors' for detecting pain. He also believed that our body had its own pathway to the brain, and its own area of the brain for processing pain signals, but this has since been proved to be incorrect.

It's true to say that there are still some doctors who apply this theory to chronic pain, as it falls in line with the thinking, that if we remove the cause, then the pain will go along with it. Once again, many people who experience chronic pain will have a very different story.

Gate Control Theory

A great deal is now known about the Gate Control Theory of pain. This has been developed for over 40 years by Professor Patrick Wall of St. Thomas Hospital and Dr. Ronald Melsack of Magill University in Canada. These two medical professionals are two of the world leaders in the subject. Since this theory was first discussed, it has proved to have been a huge influence in the way the medical profession now understand the process that happens within the body of someone with chronic pain.

This Gate Control Method is included in the hypnosis and visualisation element of my Pain Management Program to help people relieve pain, so let's explain more about it.

The theory suggests that there is a neural mechanism in the spinal cord which acts like a gate, which can increase or decrease the flow of nerve impulses from surface fibres to the central nervous system. It involves the interaction between what are called T-cells and small and large fibres that can either increase or decrease the pain signal moving up the spinal cord. In this way, sometimes the signal never reaches the brain. The greater the level of pain stimulation, the 'gate' is less able to block it from the brain.

When the amount of information passing through the gate goes over a critical level, it activates the neural areas responsible for the pain experience and the response. So according to gate control theory, we have a series of these pain control gates situated in the spinal cord, and at the base of the brain. These can be fully open depending on certain factors, or completely closed.

So if we experience anxiety, fear, apprehension or depression; in other words, messages coming down from the brain, the 'suffering' aspect of pain; then these gates are fully opened. By contrast, if a person feels relaxed and content, those gates can be partially or completely closed to exclude much or all of that pain. This also explains why those people who are hypnotised or distracted in some way may not even notice the injury or the normal pain associated with it.

If there is a lot of information coming into the surface fibres, such as touching the skin, rubbing or light scratching, and then these fibres can close the gate and stop the perception of pain, as it is not viewed as a danger to the body. This probably explains why heat and cold treatments, and massage are very good for reducing pain.

When I was a child we would attach clothes pegs to the skin on our arms to see who could stand the discomfort the longest. It really is surprising how the pain subsided the longer the peg was left in place. It was the brain registering that the discomfort was not life threatening and therefore, it became almost imperceptible over time. By the time a pain messenger reaches the brain, it is either reduced to a low level or entirely eliminated.

You will learn the techniques that enable you to control the level of information passing through those gates, to close those gates down and therefore reduce or eliminate the experience of pain, and letting your body create its own feelings of comfort anytime you want it. No clothes pegs involved, honest.

There are 3 factors which influence the 'opening and closing' of these gates.

Here are several factors that Melzack said can open the gate:

- Physical factors; such as injury or activation of the large fibres
- Emotional factors; such as anxiety, worry, tension and depression
- Behavioural factors; such as focusing on the pain or boredom.

This gate control theory also suggests that certain factors close the gate.

- Physical factors, such as medication, stimulation of the small fibres
- Emotional factors, such as happiness, optimism or relaxation
- Behavioural factors, such as concentration, distraction or involvement in other activities.

These mental techniques are known as self-hypnosis. This method differs from many others you may have used before. It is almost certain that you have been to see a GP or pharmacist to discuss your pain and received drugs designed to help.

If you have not, then it is essential that you do so before using the techniques, or listening to any recordings that you will be able to access, once you have read this book. These techniques are not a substitute for professional medical diagnosis of any pain you experience.

Once you have done this, and both you and your medical practitioner are satisfied regarding the cause of the pain symptoms, this method may well help you to take some control.

9. Your New Prescription

Hypnosis and Meditation

There are so many misconceptions regarding hypnosis, that it is really important for you to understand a few things before you even consider using Self Hypnosis to help yourself manage Chronic Pain.

When you ask most people what hypnosis is usually used for, the answers range from the extreme and blatantly untrue, (controlling others, making them do what you want) or make them look stupid to give you a laugh on stage, to stop smoking, and helping to lose weight.

The truth is that hypnosis was first used for healing as early as 500 BC by the Egyptians. It was used in the Greek Sleep Temples, by the Hebrews for meditation, and with breathing exercises and meditation. The Buddhist tradition used darkened rooms with music and chanting to get to this altered state, and of course the American Indians had Shaman.

You will have heard the term to be "Mesmerised" and this word comes from the man himself, Anton Mesmer who in 1771 developed the theory of Animal Magnetism and Magnetic Fluid in the body. His techniques were used by many people to great effect and began the investigations into the workings of the mind as a means of healing the body.

Others followed in Mesmers footsteps and one notable Surgeon, James Esdaile, used Mesmerism in India during the 1800's where he performed 300 major operations, and 3000 minor operations, using pure suggestion as the means of anaesthesia. Bringing the mortality rate down from almost 80% to 8%

It was a Scottish surgeon, James Braid, who became known as the 'father of hypnosis' when he named it such from the Greek word 'Hypnos' which means 'sleep'. However, as many people who have experienced formal hypnosis will testify, the participant is not asleep; they simply look as if they are.

James Braid, used Hypnosis during surgery, and for helping people heal from many physical ailments. As you can see; it's true to say that Hypnosis has been used medically since time began.

Hypnosis is a state of heightened awareness and focused concentration; (Spegal & Bloom 1983)

It is 'a state of inner absorption, concentration, and focused attention. It is like using a magnifying glass to focus the rays of the sun and make them more powerful. Hypnosis allows people to use more of their potential, learning self-hypnosis is the ultimate act of self-control.' (American Society of Clinical Hypnosis)

It is these self-same techniques that you can access and use, after reading this book, to help yourself manage Chronic Pain. My self-help pain management programme is all you will need to put what you have read here, into practice and begin to see the results for yourself.

Hypnosis enables you to focus attention on achieving the positive healthy outcome that is most important to you, and move you away from the experience of pain. Hypnosis is purely and simply focused, concentrated attention on a concept or an idea. We use hypnosis to focus on the solution rather than the problem.

Throughout your life, before you ever experienced this pain, your body has built up a whole host of physical and psychological experiences, of healthy function, which means you are able to control and even eliminate your level of discomfort. Your subconscious mind, has all of these memories stored, so that you have an infinite resource of powerful memories of what your life was like before your health problems appeared. These memories go all the way back to your baby years, to toddler years, of running around walking, skipping, jumping and climbing. The fun and interesting places you visited and the things you did.

During all of these years, during which your body enjoyed good health, strength, energy and comfort, your mind, has all of these memories stored within your subconscious and because they are still there, you can get to them.

You can remember many times I'm sure, when you have been focused on something other than the pain, that you were completely unaware of it. It's as if you temporarily forgot you had pain, until your attention is once again brought back to it. The pain is just not experienced, does it actually go away? or is there something else going on? Something that our body does? Something that our mind does?

What is going on when a parent has a severe migraine headache, where it feels totally debilitating, however the moment their child is hurt or in some kind of danger, they immediately take action, and their own pain disappears. There are so many times in everyday life where I'm sure you have noticed that the pain you experience, simply disappears as you go about your day, you simply forget to notice it.

In your own life before you developed this pain, your body was healthy and strong. As your mind recalls these feelings of comfort and wellbeing, your body is able to once again re-experience these feelings; using them as a focus of attention. You direct your mind, your thoughts away from the problems and onto the solution. Even people with chronic pain can do this. People who have cancer are taught to help themselves alleviate the pain of their condition with the deep hypnotic relaxation methods used in hypnosis.

Hypnosis for pain control simply uses the natural ability that you already possess, to aneasthetise and create a form of amnesia towards the pain sensations. To focus on something else, so that the discomfort you have been feeling is simply forgotten.

Without question, all medical professionals are dedicated people, working hard to help you to the best of their ability, with the resources they have, and in the confines of regulation. But many conventional treatments in the western world tend to focus on the illness. They focus on the problem, then the diagnosis, rather than focusing on where you want to get to.

It's safe to say that no medical professional is trained in hypnosis as part of their medical qualification. Very few, are sufficiently trained in the use of hypnosis after they have qualified as GP's. Those who are interested in qualifying as a Hypnotherapist have to pay privately for this training, and even then, it may not be something that they are allowed to use within their practice, within the United Kingdom's National Health Service system. (NHS). Therefore they are unable to use it or recommend it to their patients. Another reason for the NHS being reluctant to recommend hypnosis, is due to the differing levels of expertise and the unregulated nature of the profession.

In fact, the power of the mind is brushed over within the training of our medical professionals, even though it is recognised that it plays a role in our ability to heal. It takes a shift away from looking at the illness, and focusing instead on the health of the client or patient in order to get results from the use of Hypnosis.

One important factor to be aware of with this approach is to understand that, the subconscious mind finds it difficult to deal with negatives. It is imperative to use positive-focused language.

If someone says to you; "Don't think of a pink elephant", or a blue sky; you immediately think of that pink elephant or that blue sky. This is because the word 'don't' is a negative word and the subconscious fails to recognise it. You immediately get the image of a pink elephant or blue sky, so that your subconscious has a clear image of what you have asked it not to do. It needs this image in order for it to follow your instruction.

However, as you can see, by the time it has identified what a pink elephant looks like or what a blue sky is, your subconscious has already thought about it. You get the opposite effect of what you wanted.

You will always get more of what you focus on. Think again about what you DO want to achieve and you will have far more success than focusing on what you want to avoid.

If you get into a taxi and tell the driver you don't want to go to the airport, will that get you to where you want to go? Of course not! You have to tell the driver where you DO want to go, not where you don't want to go. The same thing applies to your mind. Tell your mind what you want to achieve and it will open the doorway to the various pathways to achieving that goal. When you create a positive vision on the positive outcome you want to achieve, by focusing on that representation, and by taking all the steps necessary to make this representation a daily reality, you will not only be responding to a problem but also creating a solution; Your very own solution.

One single footstep will not create a pathway. You have to keep treading the same ground over and over again to create a pathway. Similarly, a single thought will not create a pathway in your mind. You have to think and think the same thoughts to create that mental, or neural pathway. That is why the self-hypnosis techniques are practiced daily to find the relief you want.

In the same way your doctor will prescribe antibiotic drugs to be taken for a certain length of time. You are told to finish the course or your illness will return. Your self-hypnosis is your own self-prescribed daily treatment, without the added side effects associated with many drugs.

Using self-hypnosis in this way, you are also becoming an active participant in your own healing and recovery. Take the initiative and you will be actively making your success happen, and making it a daily reality in your life. You will be actively engaged in creating the health, comfort and wellbeing your body needs. It will be very different from anything you may have done before. In order to create change, we have to do something different, when all our usual avenues have been explored.

In all likelihood you have taken one medicine after another, and waited to see what happens. Maybe waiting many weeks for lab test results, or visiting one specialist after another, waiting for the second opinion, maybe even the third and even fourth opinions. Maybe, and it is quite likely, that up until now, you have been rather passive in the whole process; waiting to receive the cure, and the outcome of other people's action and intervention.

This process is different, with hypnosis; you are the specialist on yourself. You hold the full knowledge of your own life, your inner feelings and emotions and the resources deep inside you, which you can mobilise to achieve the result you want; Health, wellbeing and calmness.

You are going to be actively involved in making your success happen. If you have any doubts right now, that you do indeed have the ability to make it happen, that's ok. These doubts will be turned on their heads, when you begin to see the benefits, and this will lead to optimism, and eventual certainty, that this is working for you. The benefits will turn into a daily reality.

When you truly hold on to the certainty, that you already have all the resources that you need to recover, you will recover. When you have the certainty that you can control and manage the pain, so you have a much better experience of daily life, then that is exactly what you will get. If we actively create that wellbeing, then what is happening here is that you set up a very powerful expectation; this in itself will become the self-fulfilling prophecy.

During the process of doing self-hypnosis, I am going to presume that you will enjoy the success you want to have. Building in certainty that you are going to rid yourself of that old burden of pain and replace it with feelings of wellbeing, it is an objective fact, a certainty, that you already have the resources in you to make your future of bodily wellbeing a reality.

From the previous discussion, you, like all living things, have those inner 'unseen influences' that are an inherent part of all biological life. All we are doing here is showing you how to get to them, so that you can use them for your benefit.

There are a variety of ways that you can get the comfort and relief you want. If you decide to use hypnosis and meditation to help yourself, you will be shown these different ways, because no single approach will be helpful for everyone in the same way. Just as no one else's pain experience is the same as yours. Some of the techniques will connect with you immediately, others may not. You will find the ones that do connect powerfully with your own experience, and you can use them again and again, letting your mind, learn and respond in the way that is right for you.

You need to actively participate. This is the key to enabling you to get relief quickly and easily. Let's look at what you will be doing when you decide to use my Self-Help programme or decide to have 1:1 sessions;

I'm sure there have been many times in your life where you have become so intently absorbed in something you were doing. Something that captured your imagination and attention so much, that everything else around you was blocked out of your conscious awareness. Maybe it was reading a book, watching a film, being at the theatre, watching a play. It almost feels as if you are part of the story. Maybe it is singing, dancing, acting or something else that you got so involved in, it became real to you. Some people have spiritual experiences, whether it was part of some organised movement or not.

Maybe you have been involved in exploring a new place, or fascinated by being out in the countryside. Have you ever been so involved in your favourite sport or engrossed in your hobby that it has taken up all your focused attention? There must have been countless times in your life where you have experienced these creative flows of energy. It is that same kind of intense imaginative involvement that you will learn to experience. Active experience of getting your body healthy, well and comfortable, and because you want this sense of real comfort, you will find it far easier than you imagined.

These methods work best when they are simply allowed to happen, without insistence or demand on your part. Without putting yourself under pressure to feel or experience certain things. This process puts you back into a position of action rather than dependency on chemicals that quite often stop working as effectively as they once did.

Many people often need stronger and stronger doses of a drug for it to give them the same effect and the relief they need. You will be more proactive, more in tune with your body and its responses, and more able to use these responses, and direct them in a way that is right for you. You will move away from being the passive victim where you feel out of control, and as you gain more skill with this process, you will feel increasingly in charge; Creating step by step, a future free from pain and full of comfort.

We are all born with the potential to achieve everything that we want to achieve in life. Yet as we grow up we are subjected to ways of thinking and ways of doing which are useful in one situation, but then become a problem when we move to a different situation in life. The great thing is that the unconscious part of the mind has the power to learn differently.

Our brain has something called 'Plasticity', simply put; it means we can teach it new tricks. Hypnosis helps to focus on the outcome you want. Focus creates reality and you can use the language of the subconscious mind to power you forward into feeling more in charge of yourself, and responding rather than reacting and resisting what is. This gives us more choices, so that we have more new and useful ways of dealing with new situations.

Mindfulness Meditation - Benefits and Side Effects

Along with hypnosis, the use of mindfulness meditation is another very powerful way of managing Chronic Pain. Mindfulness was teamed with cognitive therapy and is a treatment that was originally developed by Professor Mark Williams at the University of Toronto. The primary aim was to help people who suffered recurring episodes of depression due to other illnesses. After lengthy studies, Mindfulness Based Cognitive Therapy (MBCT) was found to be as effective as antidepressants, with none of the harmful side effects. It is so effective; it is now recognised in the UK by the National Institute of Clinical Excellence (NICE) as the preferred treatment for depression.

Many conditions and illnesses that result in pain for patients can also result, and often does result, in feelings of anxiety and depression, due to the feelings of being out of control of the pain itself. MBCT works on these feelings of stress, anxiety and depression and also on the experience of pain itself.

To help you to understand that mindfulness meditation is a valid therapeutic tool for pain, I want to outline some of the studies and research. In this way, you can fully understand the benefits to you, so that you can apply them to yourself using the methods I use with my pain-management clients. Experiments have been conducted on the effects of Meditation and the experience of pain. Three experiments were conducted to measure pain-sensitivity, and the actual rating of the pain on a numerical scale.

Participants in the experiment were taught to use meditation and they were given 3 days of meditation for 20 minutes each day. Their pain-ratings and sensitivity were rated before and after the experiments. The findings showed that the use of mindfulness meditations reduce pain and anxiety.

The meditations 'analgesic effects' are related to reduced anxiety and on the patients enhanced ability to focus on the present moment. (Journal of Pain - March 2010)

When practiced daily; overtime mindfulness brings long term changes in your mood and in your levels of happiness and wellbeing, and a significant reduction in the pain sensations. The scientific studies have shown that mindfulness not only prevents anxiety and depression, but it also positively affects the brain patterns underlying day to day anxiety, stress, depression, and irritability, so that if and when they do arise, they dissolve away again far more easily. Other studies have also shown that people who meditate regularly, see their doctors less often and spend fewer days in hospital.

Meditation has been used for centuries as a spiritual practice performed by people from other cultures. Meditation is not a religion. It is simply a method of training the mind, and it has been used successfully to treat depression, anxiety, stress and to lower blood pressure. Many people who practice meditation are religious, but there are many atheists and agnostics who meditate too.

Meditation need not take too much of your time, 5 minutes to start with is fine, and then it can be increased to 20 minutes or more per day. If pain is stopping you from doing things and from being active, you can use this time to practice meditation, and free your time so you have more of it to spend on the things you want.

Meditation needs your active participation and persistence and you can be taught quite easily to do this. You can work with me 1:1 or by using my Self-Help Pain Management Program. This program is a more in-depth step by step guide to the strategies and techniques spoken of here, and offered as bonuses with this book. They provide you with all you need to bring comfort to both your mind and body. What have you got to lose?

When you decide to use Hypnosis and Meditation to help control pain, your therapist will take you through a set of questions to get a clear picture of your issues, and they will also take note of some of your history. This includes an in-depth assessment of the pain you experience. You are likely to be asked where it's located, how long it lasts, how intense it is, how often you get the pain, does it lessen or worsen at various times. You will be asked to describe it as best you can, and if you notice what triggers it and what makes the pain worse or better.

You will also be asked about the emotions, thoughts, and behaviors you have when in pain. What are your personal coping strategies, what are your physical limitations, and any other consequences of pain, such as; limitations, financial problems, social, and so on.

It is always imperative that a medical diagnosis has been given for the continuance of pain, because there may well be an underlying cause, and most hypnotherapists are not medically qualified. Your therapist will therefore take your medical/health history including how the pain began, and what types of treatments have you received for pain, including any medication prescribed. They will more than likely contact your GP to keep him/her informed and to ask if there is any known reason why hypnosis or meditation would not be recommended.

Therapy sessions are designed to help you cope with pain and to bring an easiness into your life. Sessions will teach you to think more realistically about the pain and other things in your life. Pain Management therapy helps you to relax much more than before, by using deep breathing techniques and relaxation exercises, to help you to pace your daily activities so that you are not feeling that you do too much on 'good' days and very little on 'bad' days, which only serve to perpetuate the cycle of negative thinking.

Once you become more focused in these areas and begin to feel the benefits, it also allows you to be much more assertive in how you communicate with others in your life, and that includes your GP or other medical professionals, family and friends, helping you to solve problems related to the pain you experience, and the other stresses in your life.

The sessions offered in my practice involve cognitive-behavioral strategies too, and these start by focusing on the management of pain, and then moves to other issues. The main aim here is to change any negative, unrealistic thoughts, images, and beliefs about the pain, and the consequences of having pain. This will also help you to identify certain behaviours that may worsen the pain for you, so that you can learn new coping strategies as well as become more adaptable. Most people can feel better after 6-8 sessions practicing diligently over 12-16 weeks.

People who seek cognitive therapy for pain management are often seeking medical care for their pain as well. As a result, many people are prescribed medications to assist with pain management. Medication is prescribed based on the diagnosis of the pain problem as well as the severity of pain experienced. For mild to moderate pain, most medical professionals prescribe non-opioid medications, or non-steroidal anti-inflammatory drugs such as ibuprofen, or Naproxen. However, many more people are prescribed extremely strong drugs, whose side effects can cause more problems than the pain itself.

Although many people become very skilled using Hypnosis and Meditation, and these people have found they can stop using painkilling drugs, it is not always a substitute for pain medication, for those who experience chronic pain. However, it can, and is used alongside a client's usual medication. After starting a programme of Hypnosis and Meditation in this way, many clients do report that they are using far less medication as the sessions progress, and that has to be a good thing.

10.Conclusion

For most of my adult life I suffered from severe migraine attacks every single month, sometimes more than this. Each time I had a migraine attack it would put me out of action for at least four days. For those who have regular migraine attacks, you will likely have some understanding of the level of pain. As I mentioned in the introduction, we all experience pain uniquely. However, the effects of the acute pain sensations, the nausea and vomiting, visual disturbances and the total draining effect on energy leaves, many migraine sufferers like me, feel like a wet rag for the whole length of the attack.

The effect on my working life was pretty difficult as it meant many absences from work, and the added consequences were the increased levels of stress this brought into my life, and needless to say, more migraine episodes. It was a real vicious cycle of stress, pain, muscle tension, and over-reliance on the drugs that vary rarely did much to ease my condition. I began taking a prescribed drug for migraine over 30 years ago and I have to say, that really helped to shift the migraine rather quickly, however, once the effect of the drug wore off I would take another.

Over a period of four days per month, I would wake with a migraine, take a pill, have relief for much of the day, the pain would return and I would take another pill to get me through the night. The pills didn't stop the attacks from coming each month, but they did help me to have less time off work and get through the days. If the pill didn't shift the pain for that particular attack, on occasion I was left once again to suffer the pain as I could only take one pill in 24hrs.

I also suffered with the side effects from these drugs, tiredness, tightness in my throat and weakness in my arms and legs. Pretty heavy stuff to endure simply to get rid of a 'headache' and this went on for almost 15 years of my life!

I decided to look at what else I could do to help myself, and I began looking into the use of meditation as a form of relaxation. This coincided with undertaking my degree at Northumbria University. I have always had a fascination for how the mind works and how our thoughts influence our reality. The more I learnt, the more I practiced and the calmer I became. The results were amazing and the migraine attacks became less frequent and more manageable.

Following my degree and my work with a mental health charity, I decided to look further into hypnosis and I was hooked. Combining Hypnosis and Meditation, I find that my body responds in the way I want. My thoughts and emotions have shifted, from being ones of resistance, to ones of allowing. I realised the more tense I became, the more I fought against the pain, the more pain I experienced. At first it wasn't easy to practice the meditation or use the hypnosis when the pain was severe.

As with learning anything new, I had to be persistent and consistent in my approach. I wanted to perfect the techniques and I found the best way to incorporate hypnosis and meditation into my life was to use it when I was actually migraine free, to make it part of my daily routine, and I have felt the benefits and continue to feel the benefits of hypnosis and meditation on my own body ever since.

Recently a client of mine was having a skype session with me. She told me from the outset that this particular morning she was in the midst of a migraine attack, and had considered cancelling her session. I congratulated her on having the courage to go ahead, because not only was she breaking the negative pattern of giving into the pain and keeping the negative cycle going, but she could also strengthen her belief in the power of the techniques she was learning.

The session went ahead and at the end when I asked her how she was feeling, she told me the migraine had gone. What better way to experience the power of your own mind. Would she have regretted going back to bed? You bet. Would she have worried about the missed day and the work not getting done with its missed deadlines? Of course!

The repercussion for her would have meant a continuation of the 'old' coping strategies and maintaining a cycle of pain that she was wishing to break. We live in an instant response mentality, the 'pill for all ills society', we want a quick and easy cure for everything. What we lose with this approach is the knowledge of our own powerful resources, and skills. We essentially are de-skilling ourselves. We have forgotten how to use our own healing processes and have become dependent on outside influences to give us the life we want.

What I wanted to do with this book was to bring together information and knowledge, research and science, to help you to understand that YOU can relieve pain, and often eliminate it, simply by using the god-given resources of the miracle that is your mind and body.

Yes it will take some time and a little input from yourself, it will take your belief in your abilities, and it will take courage to step up and do something differently. There is a saying that goes something like this: *"If you always do what you've always done, you will always get what you've always got"*. So if you want a different result, be prepared, and willing to do something differently.

Using the information in this book, practicing the techniques from the free bonuses that come with it; Using the full self-help programme that I have put together for you, I can guarantee that with persistent, and consistent application, you will also benefit as I have, and as many of my clients have, and re-gain that level of control over your life once again.

Many of my clients use the self-help programme along with 1:1 sessions to reinforce it, and to address certain changes with their condition. If this is something you feel would benefit you, then you can contact me to discuss the way forward for you.

This self-help programme is designed to be used in conjunction with any pain medication you are currently prescribed. It is important that you consult your

medical practitioner for a full diagnosis of any pain you experience and always consult your GP to discuss reducing or stopping any medication you have been given for pain, before embarking on this programme. This book, along with the self-help programme, may be something you wish to discuss with your GP as an option to helping you reduce the drugs and the related side effects.

I wanted to write this book to help you understand that the way you think, has a powerful impact on your experience.

We always get more of what we focus on. Our focus does indeed create our reality. Are you going to continue to focus on the negative experience of pain, or do you choose now, to take a different path and focus on the peaceful mind and body that you truly want? What's it to be?

Appendix:

References have been made throughout this book from the following sources:

Ader. R. (1981) Psychoneuroimmunology

BinauralBeats.com

British Medical Journal (1995)

Birch.V. (2008) Living well with Pain and Illness

Chapman.R. & Bonica.J. (1985) Intractable Pain

Discovery Health Channel (2003) Placebo. Mind over Medicine.

Esdaile. J. (1846) Hypnosis in Medicine and Surgery. New York: Julien Press

Goodmam. R. & Blank.M. (2006) Journal of Cellular Psychology

Horgan.J. (1999) The Undiscovered Mind

Jemmer.P. Northumbria University UK

Kirsch et al (2002) American Psychological Association. Article 23

Lozanov, Georgi. (2006) Suggestology and Suggestopedy.

Lipton.B.H. (2005) Biology of Belief

Mason.A.A. (1952) British Medical Journal 30 442-443

McClare.C.W.F. (1974) Resonance in Biogenetics

Mosely.J.B. O'Malley.K (2002) New England Journal of Medicine

Myss.C. (1997) Why People Don't Heal and How They Can

NLP LearningSystems.com

Pert.C. (1986) Brain/Mind Bulletin

Pert.C. (1997) Molecules of Emotion

Spiegel.D. & Bloom JR (1983) Group Therapy and Hypnosis Metastatic Breast Carcinoma Pain.

Turk. D.C. Meichenbaum.D. & Genest.M (1983) Pain and Behavioral Medicine

Wall.P. & Melzack. R (1965) Gate Control Theory of Pain

Zeidan.F et al (2010) Journal of Pain Vol.11 Issue 3

Thank You

I do hope you enjoyed the contents of this book, and indeed recommend to others that may be experiencing Pain on a daily basis, and believe there is an alternative to drugs in order to become well.

A link to purchase further copies may be found at the main website; www.SubconsciousMedicine.com

You may download your bonuses at the secret link here; www.SubconsciousMedicine.com/bonuses

Dee Twentyman BsC.(hons),DHP, MAPHP(Acc.) CNHC